# Perimenopause Please

# Perimenopause Please

✦

## The Psychological Impact of Perimenopause

*Nancy L. Whelan, R.N., M.S., M.S.*

iUniverse, Inc.
New York  Lincoln  Shanghai

# Perimenopause Please
## The Psychological Impact of Perimenopause

iUniverse books may be ordered through booksellers or by contacting:

iUniverse
2021 Pine Lake Road, Suite 100
Lincoln, NE 68512
www.iuniverse.com
1-800-Authors (1-800-288-4677)

ISBN-13: 978-0-595-34624-0 (pbk)
ISBN-13: 978-0-595-79370-9 (ebk)
ISBN-10: 0-595-34624-3 (pbk)
ISBN-10: 0-595-79370-3 (ebk)

Printed in the United States of America

I would like to dedicate this book to J$^3$.

# Contents

# *Preface*

The very foundation of this book originated due to the *pervasive* lack of open and meaningful communication between women about the process of perimenopause. What was perimenopause anyway? I really wasn't *that* familiar with the term until it became personal. I discovered that perimenopause is the time frame "surrounding" a woman's last menstrual period (or menopause).[1] Upon entering perimenopause myself, I discovered that women were quite hesitant discussing their own unique experiences with perimenopause. When they *did* talk about it, the information they shared was vague and there seemed to be an undercurrent of different emotions from embarrassment, ill feelings, anger, and even denial. Since other women weren't talking to me about perimenopause, and I really didn't know what to expect, I embarked on a quest to gather as *much* written information as I could to better understand the entire perimenopause process. Subsequently, during my information gathering endeavor, and to my complete surprise, I became very aware of the fact that there was little written material available on the psychological impact of perimenopause. I knew that the cerebral aspect of the entire perimenopause progression *had* to be *extremely* important because of the cognitive changes that were happening to me and because of the different emotions that I was experiencing. And, it became glaringly evident to me that there was not only an enormous communication gap that existed *between* women, but there was also a severe *lack of information* offered in the written psychological realm concerning perimenopause.

By the conclusion of this project, I was amazed at how much there really was to learn about perimenopause. For instance, did you know that in America eighty percent of women will experience some negative perimenopausal signs? Or, were you aware that after menopause approximately a third of women will experience a decreased sex drive? Or, did you know that two thirds of the domestic violence in women aged 45 and over is female violence directed toward the male? Or, did you know that after the menopausal transition, most women feel better overall? As you read on, you will be as surprised as I was at how much there is to know about perimenopause.

Furthermore, because of a *very* negative overall perception that still exists in this society concerning the menopause process, this book explores the evolvement of that general negativity and what can be done by women today, and even society as a whole, to conquer this pessimism that is nothing short of passé and actually quite harmful to women. Women will learn how to enthusiastically anticipate and gracefully receive the positive elements of this time of life, therefore, the personal gains, development, growth, and freedom that they will experience during perimenopause (menopause and post menopause) and women will also learn how to openly accept and manage the negative elements of this time of life, therefore, the unpleasant physical/psychological signs, the inconveniences, and other mid-life events that may also be occurring at the same time. The very title of the book is dichotomous in that: (1) It suggests this enthusiasm and anticipation that every woman should embrace: *Please let perimenopause enter my life, I am ready for it!* And (2), the title also reflects the break-down in communication between women: *Please tell me more about perimenopause. I really need to know!*

This book was designed to document my own personal journey through perimenopause so that other women would not have to proceed through their own perimenopause without a personal narrative from someone else to help them along. Sometimes it helps knowing that someone else is experiencing similar feelings, signs, and/or events. And, since the mid-life experience is also occurring during this particular time in the lifespan, you will learn how men experience the same peripheral, significant mid-life events as women. You will find this book quite unique in that I concentrate on the psychological elements of perimenopause and *not* the numerous physiological elements of perimenopause that so much of the current literature emphasizes.

# 1

# *Introduction*

*What is happening to me?* I wondered, stretching for the car door handle attempting to close the door. The recurrent joint aches in my wrists and my elbows were really starting to become an annoyance. Struggling to shut the car door with a sore wrist, I remembered the song *Haven't got time for the pain.* Maybe there really was something to that song. Carly Simon must have known something so many years ago, that was only now becoming very clear to me. Pain was an inconvenience. The joint trouble I was experiencing lately was somewhat ambiguous, nondescript, and intermittent making it more of a nuisance than anything else. Every time I thought I should visit a doctor, the pain would disappear as quickly as it had appeared, and I never would make it to the doctor. Some days the joint pain didn't bother me at all.

*Maybe I'm developing carpal tunnel syndrome that everyone seems to be getting lately.* I silently contemplated. But, if in fact I was suffering from carpal tunnel, that didn't explain the elbow aches. I didn't play tennis, swim, or participate in any other activity that might trigger elbow pain. And…I was not engaging in any repetitive motion that might trigger a carpal problem. It was all a mystery to me.

"So, what's the matter?" I caught myself asking out loud. The joint trouble and numerous other problems that had recently been affecting me were actually quite insidious, yet as subtle as the little nuisances were, the physical and psychological consequences would soon prove to be life-moving.

Listening to the car stereo, my upper body moving to the rhythm, my mind wandered. I recognized that in addition to the joint aches I was experiencing, there were actually *many* changes that had been affecting me on many different levels lately. In fact, some physical changes had started occurring a couple of years prior to my 45th birthday, but this 45th year saw the most marked alterations. Not only were there outward visible signs of what was happening to my physical body, but there were internal, emotional changes taking place as well.

*How old am I now?* I asked myself, mulling my chronological age over in my mind. *Forty-five*. Suddenly I realized the implications of a woman approaching middle age—menopause! And, here *I* was in middle age. Truthfully, I was fed up with the entire reproductive nonsense anyway. I had one twelve year old son and I didn't want any more children. I was also worn out from the monthly inconveniences and disruptions. I had heard somewhere in my travels that when a woman had reached the point in her life when she was *completely* disgusted with and totally over the reproductive cycle, she was approaching "the change". Of course, any woman of any age, including myself, would experience occasional frustration and displeasure with the reproductive cycle throughout the years, but my intense discontent had never reached this level of dissatisfaction until now. And, while driving my car that sun-drenched Florida morning, I knew that I was entering another chapter in my life. As much as I feared it, strangely enough, I welcomed it. I felt that I was ready for what life had to offer me next even though I knew little about the road ahead.

Acknowledging that my journey into mid-life was truly beginning, I wanted to learn as much about "the change" as possible. I wanted to hear first-hand from other women who had experienced the conclusion of their childbearing years. So…I set out to gather as many stories as I could about the menopause process. It was funny though, because *many* of the slightly older women, as well as the much older women I knew, who had already experienced what I was about to experience, apparently did *not* like talking about the "change". I zealously tried to solicit any information on the subject that I could get from others to help me better understand and willingly accept the transformation, but any discussion about it would invariably be redirected to another topic, or the woman would give absolutely *no* valuable information whatsoever, leaving me in the dark still.

"Oh, nothing really happened to me," one friend explained.

"Everyone makes too much of it," said another.

"I didn't realize there was a name for it," one acquaintance replied when I casually mentioned to her one day that I was having a "perimenopausal moment". Like me, before researching this book, she was unaware of the term "perimenopause". And, she later shared with me that she too was experiencing similar perimenopausal signs such as forgetfulness and overall doldrums, yet she did not realize that there was a process with a name that prefaced menopause.

"That seemed like such a long time ago, I really can't remember what happened," an eighty-something-year-old family member clarified to me.

*Wow!* I thought. It is really great that the changes these women experienced during the menopause transition were so understated, but I didn't believe a word *any* of them were saying. There had to be *some* changes somewhere along the line that they had experienced and remembered that they could share with me. Or…maybe they just weren't sharing! From their tone of voice and the obvious lack of content in what they were actually revealing to me, I was left with the impression that there may have been some embarrassment, ill feelings, anger, and even denial! I was getting absolutely *no* helpful information on the topic whatsoever from women I was acquainted with. And one day, I suddenly realized that some of the feelings these women were displaying—anger, denial, and shame—were the *exact* same feelings one experiences in the grieving process. I remembered learning about these same emotions in one of Elisabeth Kubler-Ross's[2] books on the grieving process. Furthermore, a feeling of isolation and depression were two more stages that had been theorized in the grieving process, and I was experiencing *both* of these emotions lately. I was feeling very alone in this life experience, and the fact that people were unwilling to share their experiences with me removed me even further from the humanness and relational part of the whole "change" thing that women go through.

*Was menopause a grieving process?* I wondered. There were definitely losses involved to some degree. At the time of menopause, there was a loss of the ability to bear children, a loss of some physical wellness, and most importantly a loss of female hormones, most notably estrogen. It amazed me how one hormone like estrogen, or lack of it, could wreak so much havoc in a woman's life.

A couple of the women I appealed to for information had the unfortunate experience of undergoing surgical menopause. Because of the surgical removal of their ovaries, they were immediately thrust into a situation that was very different than anything they had ever experienced before—instantaneous menopause. Even though many of the signs they had were similar to that of natural menopause, they were placed on hormone therapy (HT) almost immediately post-op which made the entire process distinct for them, making it difficult for me to totally relate to their menopause experience. However, I should mention that this group of surgically-induced menopausal women seemed to share their personal stories with me much more freely than the naturally menopausal women I spoke with.

From my conversations with menopausal and post-menopausal women, naturally menopausal, and surgically-induced menopausal women, it became very apparent to me that there was a *tremendous* gap in the information that was being shared between women, for one reason or another, who were exiting or had already exited their childbearing years. It probably would have made my understanding much clearer right from the beginning, when I first began investigating the process, if others had communicated their familiarity with this evolving nature of events without restraint. This lack of frank female expression was quite puzzling to me, and rendered me almost devoid of knowledge on the topic that I had enthusiastically looked for and counted on.

I pleasantly reminisced back to the time my son was born twelve years earlier. There had been *no* problems whatsoever receiving narratives from other women, who were *more* than willing to share their stories about their newborn babies. In fact, they would divulge things to me without me ever having to ask! Women (whether I knew them or not) would come right up to me when I was obviously very pregnant and they would start rattling off things I never would have dreamed they would reveal to me. Anyway, there is a special female bond about being pregnant and having a baby. An unspoken female connection of, "Oh yes, you are going through the same thing as I did," exists. It was obvious that mothers *loved* sharing stories with each other. Other mothers-to-be, new mothers, not so new mothers, grandmothers, great-grandmothers, godmothers—a variety of mothers shared their stories with me. And, it didn't matter what her age was either. Information flowed freely. I assumed that stories would be happily and readily available in the final stage of the human female reproductive cycle just as they were during the childbirth process. Was I mistaken!

You may be wondering, "She could have spoken with her doctor about perimenopause." Actually, I did discuss certain items with my gynecologist, a woman, whom I really admired. She was very willing to discuss the menopause transition with me. But, I wanted a more personal account of the perimenopause experience. So, I kept searching.

In my information gathering endeavor on perimenopause, it became apparent to me just how valuable the human story really is. I had always held the highest regard for advice and knowledge from others. Throughout each human life experience, and throughout history, we have used stories to pass on accumulated knowledge and wisdom. In fact, before writing instruments were ever invented, story telling was used solely as a form of communication to transfer information from one person/generation/group to another person/generation/group. According to Dr. Thomas H. Peake, who wrote *Healthy Aging, Healthy Treatment, The Impact of Telling Stories*, "Healthy stories give guidance about developmental needs and the nature of change."[3] Consistent with Dr. Peake, stories and story telling are remarkably important in defining one's self. Throughout our lives, from the time we are babies, we learn by hearing all sorts of stories from a variety of people including family members, friends, lovers, teachers, coworkers, etc. all sharing their experiences with us. These narratives assist us in our development throughout our lives and especially help us in understanding and accepting the aging process says Dr. Peake.

"Storytelling or story tending creates a rich tapestry that may be honoring, intimate, intriguing, drudgery, shaming, dramatic, hopeful, or renewing,"[4] Dr. Peake asserts. There is absolutely *no* replacing story telling and story tending with factual, scientific jargon that removes the human one-on-one experience component of communication.

My lack of success in tracking down first-hand, personal stories, which has always been one of the best teachers, led me to gather and acquaint myself with as much *written* information as I could about the perimenopause process. In the technologically advanced information age in which we live, data can easily be obtained from a variety of sources. Yet, in spite of having the modern conveniences and advantage of searching for information via the internet, e-books, CD-ROMs, DVDs, tapes, books, magazines, and through other information-seeking tools, story telling and first-hand narratives *still* remain an integral form of human communication. Even though the internet offers a wide range of readily available information, there is a detached component that exists there. The humanness of relating to others, "Oh yes, she is feeling the same way as I am," is somewhat removed. Personal human interaction is missing. Furthermore, I unexpectedly discovered that the libraries and book stores I visited had only some books on menopause and *hardly any* on perimenopause. And, the books they did have on the subject concentrated on the physiological aspects of menopause, not the psychological aspects, and they were *extremely* scientific, very technical, and painfully long. Many of the books were in excess of 300 pages!

*Who has time to read such lengthy volumes of material any more?* I thought to myself. I hadn't read books that educationally extensive since it was required in college.

Many of the books included diagrams, pictures, and elaborate graphs of the human female anatomy describing and illustrating the physiological changes in the menopause progression. That was all really informative and very educational, but I really didn't want another anatomy class, as I was well aware of human anatomy and physiology. It was very disappointing to find *only* clinically driven books in my research that were written parallel to a dictionary or an encyclopedia, so matter-of-fact and incredibly indifferent. Weren't there any personal perimenopause stories that I could relate to? And, what about the psychological impact of perimenopause?

Most of us would probably agree that menopause has received plenty of bad publicity. From what I had previously heard about menopause in general, there was a very negative and pessimistic undertone attached to it. One of my four brothers candidly expressed his view of the changes that happen in women, "Women rot as they age!" That statement would make *any* woman dread the inevitable!!! I had even overheard one of the male bigwigs in my organization (before I was downsized) referring to my boss, who happened to be a woman in a perimenopausal state, as an "irrational, over-responding woman". I myself had witnessed her crying on several occasions, which was less than professional for someone in her position and rank. One morning, as she was informing me that I might be downsized, *she* burst out into tears! Wasn't *I* the one who was supposed to be upset and emotional? I was the one who was losing my job. I had to agree with the male VIP, she had behaved inappropriately a number of times in front of an assortment of coworkers. Whether they were subordinates, peers, or upper management, she had displayed emotions (mostly weeping) that traditionally were not acceptable in the workplace. Several of my coworkers agreed with me that on numerous occasions the boss lady had indeed displayed sudden emotion—expressing intense feelings, raising her voice, using more hand gestures than usual, and tearfulness in front of them. I sort of empathized with my boss lady though. I knew that my time was coming too. Actually, watching the boss lady reacting the way she did was an invaluable lesson for me to *absolutely never* allow myself to behave the way she did in the work environment, as difficult as that might be—weeping and sobbing in front of others. By permitting her stirring emotions to respond to difficult situations, she lost the respect of many coworkers, especially the males. I didn't see much empathy or tolerance for her perimenopausal situation either. It became *very* apparent to me that there really was no place for perimenopause in the workplace. And, with the growing number of women in the workforce today, especially with the increasing number of women holding extremely powerful positions, perimenopause will undoubtedly be introducing itself into the work environment in record numbers, at every level, in the very near future.

In any work environment, it can be so very difficult to divorce emotion from intellect in a normal state of mind, (this will be discussed further in a future book) much less have to dissociate the two in a torrent of fluctuating hormones. From what I had observed in my boss lady's behavior, this perimenopausal condition seemed to put some women at a disadvantage, especially in a business setting, because of the overwhelming emotions the individual had to negate. It seemed that the barrage of emotions was hard to put a lid on all the time, especially in a professional environment and particularly when one was under duress.

Let's face it; the word "menopause" itself is not a marvelous sounding word. It does not conjure up feelings of excitement and exhilaration. By no means does the word denote a warm, fuzzy feeling that one would look forward to or embrace. Menopause is, in a way, sort of like childbirth. We are eager about the end product—the baby, but, most of us are *extremely* apprehensive and fearful of the actual physical process of getting the baby into the world. The end result of menopause will, no doubt, be wonderful. But, the entire menopause process is like a childbirth experience in that it is a scary, intimidating process. We just don't know how our bodies are going to react to the hormonal changes until we actually start experiencing it At any rate, if we really consider the childbirth process, the majority of us seem to get through it without much difficulty. The baby is a reward to any physical discomfort. So…if we use this simple analogy, the benefits of post menopause—an end to mood swings, monthly irritability, discomfort, cravings, weight gain, accidents, no more purchasing feminine products, and freedom from the *constant* worry about birth control—will be a reward to any physical or psychological discomforts and inconveniences of perimenopause.

This book is an attempt to describe in a fairly simple and concise format my own personal experience with the natural perimenopausal transition that is occurring to me. I wanted to share my own narrative while presenting some factual information on perimenopause in a fun and entertaining manner that was informative and not too technical I have tried to avoid a scientific perspective as much as possible, since this was such a turn-off to me while conducting my research. I didn't want the book to turn into a dictionary or encyclopedia. Sprinkling in my own personal familiarity with, and sharing my own stories should give others a personal commentary that they can relate to and hopefully connect with. I have also interspersed some factual information where necessary for explanation and clarification. "Oh, that is why I am feeling this way today, because of x, y, or z." There is a psychological emphasis in the book, since the cerebral element of perimenopause is probably *the* most significant, and has been the most overlooked, in my estimation.

Additionally, this book does not provide a framework for the treatment of particular signs a woman may be experiencing in perimenopause. I did indicate what measures worked for me. But, everyone is so unique that what worked for me may or may not work for someone else. There are presently many other materials on the market that explore perimenopausal management options including hormone therapy (HT), bioidentical hormone replacement therapy (BHRT), herb therapy, diet, exercise, and other therapies.

While investigating and gathering information for this project, I saw the term "symptom" used *numerous* times, in fact most of the time, when discussing perimenopause and menopause. The word "symptom" seems to imply that an illness or an ailment exists and I was *really* appalled to see this word used so frequently in the literature. No wonder menopause had received such a bad rap! Let's define the word "symptom". Dictionary.com[5] defines a **symptom** as "an indication of a disorder or disease". Maybe I am hauling baggage from my nursing career, but to me a "symptom" indicates that an illness, a syndrome, or a disease process is taking place, as the dictionary clearly defines. A **sign**, as defined by Dictionary.com[6] however, "is something that suggests the presence or existence of a fact, condition, or quality". Historically, the terms "sign" and "symptom" have been used interchangeably in the medical model. But, the term "sign" is a much more neutral term that merely suggests a signal or a hint of something, unlike the term "symptom" which implies that a disorder or sickness is present. After seeing the term "symptom" used *hundreds* of times in the literature describing perimenopause, I was left with the impression that perimenopause was some sort of affliction that I didn't want any part of! So, for purposes of this book, I will refer to the "**signs**" of perimenopause not the "symptoms", since *every* attempt should be made to avoid the downbeat tone and negative publicity that the menopause process has already received.

Also during the research phase for this book, I was *equally as horrified* when I came across a web site stating that menopause was a condition that was *not* contagious! And, there's more. The same web site also stated that menopause posed no risk to others. Unbelievable! Perimenopause is a naturally occurring process in a woman's lifespan like puberty, or aging, and it is *not* a disorder or a disease process that the word "symptom" in the medical model so strongly implies. Indeed, it is *not* contagious!!! While we experience a hormonal shift during puberty, I have *never* heard *anyone* refer to the *symptoms* of adolescence, even though there are physical changes, sexual development (in the opposite direction), skin changes, moodiness, social role adjustments, etc. that similarly occur during that time of life.

As you read this book, please keep in mind that even though perimenopause is a universal event that affects every woman on every continent on earth, there are slight differences from one culture to another. This will be explored later in the book.

Finally, I should mention that this book was developed not only for women entering perimenopause, but for *everyone*. I say "everyone" and not just "women" because many other individuals live with the changes that are taking place in the perimenopausal woman. Spouses, significant others, children, parents, other family members, friends, and even coworkers witness the physical changes on a daily basis, as well as watching the feelings and emotions spilling from the perimenopausal woman. Most of us have been or will be connected to someone experiencing perimenopause at some point in our lives. It is *extremely* important that others are made aware of the transformation taking place in the perimenopausal woman so that they can recognize and understand the process and offer support when and where it is needed.

# 2

# *What is Perimenopause?*
# *Part 1*

What is perimenopause anyway? I had only recently become familiar with the term as it had become personal. My nursing education covered menopause briefly, but I couldn't recall hearing the word "peri" before menopause. In defining perimenopause, it will be easier to first have an understanding of what menopause encompasses and then a definition of perimenopause will follow.

The word "menopause" is derived from the New Latin and Greek languages from the words "month" and "cause to cease". Hence, **menopause** is characterized by the natural "cessation" of "monthly" menstruation. Menopause has been referred to as the "change" when in actuality it is not just *one* "change" per se, but *many, many* "changes" that happen gradually. The major change in menopause is a cessation of menstrual periods for twelve consecutive months. Menopause is technically a day that marks the time when twelve months have passed since the last period.[7] Therefore, menopause is actually a non-event (nothing happens) that historically has been coined to include *all* of the changes leading up to, including, and following menopause. However, more recently, the entire menopause process has been delineated into three categories differentiating distinct events that include: (1) **perimenopause**—the time frame preceding menopause when hormonal fluctuations☺, declines, and signs begin, (2) **menopause**—the time when there has been a cessation of a period for twelve consecutive months, and (3) **post menopause**—the entire time frame beyond menopause. For purposes of this book, the "**reproductive years**" refers to the childbearing years, or the time frame extending from adolescence to the time of perimenopause.

Menopause is the point in a woman's lifespan at which she cannot have children naturally.[8] Most women enter menopause in their late forties or early fifties. The time of onset varies from individual to individual, but in the U.S. the average woman reaches menopause at approximately fifty one years of age. It has also been postulated that the onset of menopause has a familial component to it, i.e.

the time a mother and other immediate female relatives experience menopause will likely be the same time the woman will experience menopause. However, this theory is controversial at this time. Menopause can also occur at other times during a woman's lifetime as indicated in the following paragraphs.

Some women may enter menopause before the age of forty. This is referred to as "**premature menopause**" and it has many causes.[9] Autoimmune reactions: the immune system for some reason destroys healthy ovarian cells, i.e. lupus or rheumatoid arthritis, mumps—in a small number of women this infection can spread to the ovaries shutting them down, surgical treatment and some medical treatments such as drug therapies and/or radiation, or any other ovarian damage or infection can thrust a woman into premature menopause. If premature menopause happens naturally, i.e. menopause not caused by surgical involvement or by medical/drug treatments, etc., it is now identified as premature ovarian failure (POF).[10]

**Early menopause** is menopause that occurs before the age of forty-five[11] (this is not premature menopause) and can occur for various reasons. For instance, women who smoke have a tendency to experience an earlier menopause.[12] Lifelong depression may also lead to an early menopause. According to the Archives of General Psychiatry, women were 20% more likely to enter menopause early if they had a lifetime history of depression (depression might hinder hormone production).[13] In addition, women who live in continued economic deprivation may enter menopause early. This type of early menopause is most likely due to constant elevated stress levels, poor nutrition, and/or toxins a woman may be exposed to. These stressors may contribute to egg depletion that in turn can trigger menopause.[14]

Furthermore, researchers at Brown University School of Medicine found that **physical and/or sexual violence** might also affect the onset of menopause. For example, in their study, women who had experienced abuse in childhood had a higher follicle stimulating hormone (FSH) level (as the ovaries start to shut down, the FSH level increases). And, in women aged 36–39, adulthood abuse was related to *lower* estrogen levels. They concluded that physical and/or sexual violence most likely disrupts the neuroendocrine system☺, which can then alter the onset of menopause.

And lastly, some women may experience **surgically-induced menopause** that can occur at any age. This type of menopause is caused by surgical intervention for various reasons that affects reproductive and/or hormonal functioning.

In **surgical menopause** the following situations can occur:[15]

1. If both ovaries are surgically removed, the woman will cease menstruation and she will also lack the hormonal effects the ovaries produced, therefore, she will experience menopause abruptly after surgery.

2. If only one ovary is surgically removed, menopause will occur on time as it normally would since she still has the hormonal benefit of one functioning ovary.

3. If the uterus is removed (hysterectomy), the woman will no longer menstruate, and if both ovaries are left intact, the hormonal changes of menopause will occur around the time it would normally occur for any woman, but about 2–3 years sooner. This could be due to a disruption of blood supply to the ovaries.[16] Often, if a hysterectomy does need to be performed, the ovaries are/or an ovary is left intact and spared so that the woman maintains the benefits of hormonal functioning.

4. If the uterus *and* both of the ovaries are surgically removed, then the woman will no longer menstruate or benefit from the hormonal output of the ovaries and she will experience menopause immediately after surgery.

The **post menopause** stage is the time frame that starts *after* twelve consecutive months have passed since the last period (menopause), whether natural or induced.[17] Therefore, after menopause, a woman is usually referred to as "post menopausal" for the remainder of her lifespan.

Finally, menopause is *not* just the cessation of a monthly cycle. There is *much*, *much* more involved than just a biological end to the reproductive years. It is an interaction/blend of hormonal fluctuations/declines, physical alterations, psychological alterations, and socio-cultural☺ factors.[18]

## Interesting Menopause Trivia:

1. With the average human lifespan increasing, the modern woman will live approximately a third to half of her life beyond menopause, longer than she has ever lived beyond the point of menopause.

2. The average age of women at the onset of menopause has not changed for centuries, irrespective of the increased human lifespan.

3.  5% of women may enter early menopause due to an inherited condition of having a thousand fewer eggs than other women.

4.  Up to 80% of women experiencing menopause have *some* negative physical signs.

5.  In post menopause, women may be at a greater risk for many physical conditions associated with estrogen depletion such as heart disease, osteoporosis, and mental inconsistencies (memory interruptions, neurotransmitter production interruption, and deterioration in antioxidant properties).

6.  Most bone loss occurs within five to seven years after menopause.[19]

7.  The average woman will gain 10–12 pounds of extra weight during the menopause transition.[20]

8.  In the past, menopause and the hormonal fluctuations and/or imbalances that accompany it, have historically been disregarded or they were dealt with as a mental condition. In fact, the word "hysterical" is derived from the Greek word for "uterus". In the past, many hysterectomies were even performed as a treatment for some psychological problems. Scary!

**Perimenopause** then is the time frame *preceding* menopause. The terms "climacteric" and "pre-menopause" have historically been used to describe the time of perimenopause currently being replaced with the term "perimenopause".[21] Perimenopause therefore is a relatively new term, which is the reason I could not recall having heard it during my nursing education in the early 80's. The prefix "peri" means to "enclose" or "surround", therefore, **peri**menopause is the time "surrounding" a woman's last menstrual period.[22]

Perimenopause is quite individualistic but, the average age at the onset of perimenopause is 45–47 years of age, which means that *most* women experience perimenopause for approximately 3–6 years before actual menopause. However, perimenopause *can* occur from ten to fifteen *years* before menopause.

In perimenopause, the ovaries gradually stop producing eggs and the production of sex hormones (mainly estrogen and progesterone) declines. Ovulation (release of a monthly egg) gradually tapers off and then stops altogether. Soon, there is not enough estrogen produced in the ovaries to stimulate the lining of the uterus and menstruation stops. Estrogen production will eventually drop to about one-third of what it was during the reproductive years. Ninety percent of estrogen production during the reproductive years occurs in the ovaries, however, there is still some estrogen production taking place elsewhere in the body. After menopause, small amounts of estrogen continue to be produced in these other parts of the body. For example, the adrenal glands, the liver, and the kidneys also assist in estrogen conversion. Estrogen is also produced in fat cells. Interestingly, overweight women may actually have fewer perimenopausal signs, specifically hot flashes and osteoporosis, because fat cells are producing small amounts of estrogen.[23] Finally, a new hormonal balance (in lesser amounts) is then established after menopause.

Perimenopause is a gradual process for most women. It starts with a slight drop in hormone levels that does not initially produce any signs, and the woman is probably not even aware of the gradual nature of the process. Hormone levels continue to fluctuate and they eventually decline to where there *are* physical and psychological signs. Perimenopause then, and the signs that accompany it, are actually the body's way of adapting to these fluctuating and declining hormones.[24] In perimenopause, a monthly cycle is still present, but the cycle may be irregular and there may be secretion and/or flow changes.

With the many perimenopausal signs that a woman may experience, she may be well aware that perimenopause has approached, but if she wants quantifiable confirmation, a health care professional can identify the presence of perimenopause by reviewing her medical history, assessing any perimenopausal signs, and a blood test can verify a decline in estrogen levels, which is indicative of perimenopause. Another blood test can also determine if levels of follicle stimulating hormone (FSH) have risen. Remember that as the ovaries start to shut down, this level increases.

During the course of perimenopause, there *are* physiological forces at work, but equally as important are the psychological alterations and modifications that are also taking place. As the information in this book unfolds, it should become *very* clear to you that perimenopause is a *powerful* process that will permeate a woman's entire existence—her behavior, her feelings, her reactions, her cognitive functioning, etc. are all affected. Additionally, the psychological powers of perimenopause can be turbulent, extensive, and intense affecting a woman negatively but, at the same time, there is also an enormous opportunity for personal growth, development, and spirituality that can affect a woman positively.

Finally, a loss of eggs and a diminishing supply of sex hormones have historically been credited for initiating perimenopause as just mentioned above. However, it should also be noted that it has been postulated that changes occurring in certain areas of the **brain** are responsible for triggering perimenopause. However, further research is needed in this area to clarify this very complex subject.

## Notable Perimenopause Particulars:

1.  Nine out of ten women will experience perimenopause.[25]

2.  Approximately 70% of women either don't have perimenopausal signs, or they don't seek professional assistance.

3.  Approximately 30% of women see a healthcare provider about perimenopausal signs.

4.  Some women will have worse perimenopausal signs if they are also experiencing other emotional stress (covered later in this book).

5.  Approximately 85% of American perimenopausal women will experience "hot flashes" according to the U.S. Food and Drug Administration.

6.  A woman's heart rate can increase by 8–16 beats during a hot flash, according to the North American Menopause Society.

7.  Women are still fertile during perimenopause and can still become pregnant.

# Is Menopause Really Necessary?
# Part 2

Now that the physiological aspects of menopause have been explored, there are other analytical hypotheses that require mention. A higher level of reasoning in explaining/justifying an end to a woman's reproductive years includes the following assertions:

1. Bearing children later in life can easily place many extra demands or burdens on an aging mother. There is the added physical burden of simply carrying the child to gestation for a woman in her fifties, sixties, and up. Pregnancy requires a *huge* commitment of nine or so months and there is an *enormous* load placed on the mother's body while being pregnant, especially if multiple births are involved. The mother's body must produce more blood to nourish the fetus, therefore increasing her heart's workload. The chance of miscarriage increases with age. Gestational diabetes☺ is more common in older mothers. There is an increased risk of pregnancy-induced hypertension (PIH). Consequently, diabetes and PIH can then make the mother more susceptible to the condition known as pre-eclampsia☺. The chances that a C-section will be performed are approximately 40% higher in an older mother. And finally, with an increase in age comes an increased risk of injury or even death to the mother during the actual childbirth process itself.

However, even in light of the above mentioned risks placed on the mother, women having children at age fifty and older has steadily increased. The Centers for Disease Control and Prevention (CDC) reported that in the year 2000 there were 255 births in the U.S. to women aged 50–54, which was an increase from 174 births in 1999.[26]

2. Becoming a mother at an older age places the child at risk for birth defects.

3. Parenting at an older age adds stress and responsibilities to the woman that she may not be equipped to handle. Stamina and energy levels after fifty are *not* what they were in the twenties and thirties. A woman of say sixty might have difficulty chasing a toddler around on a daily basis.

4. A child in this day and age in our culture requires *at least* eighteen years to raise. If a woman has had her children while she is still fairly young and in good health, then she will probably remain healthy enough to rear the child until the child is able to become independent. A mother who is ill will *not* be able to parent in the way that she would have wanted to if she is dealing with an illness, disease process, or age-related condition herself.

5. Following the above mentioned #4 reason, the "Good Mother Theory" asserts that a woman can no longer become a mother after menopause because if she were to die (which historically was a much younger age), she would have to leave her child in the care of someone else/others who may not provide the sort of nurturing environment that she would have wanted the child to be raised in, and/or the caregiver may have less devotion/attachment parenting her child than she would have had.[27]

6. The "Grandmother Hypothesis" suggests that menopause frees a woman from bearing any more children so that she will be better able to contribute to the existing children's and grandchildren's welfare, thereby enhancing their survival.[28] Studies done by Hawkes established that children who had a grandmother's help were healthier, grew faster, and gained more weight than other children, however these studies were conducted on a limited sample.[29]

7. An end to childbearing capability allows a woman to enjoy her retirement years without the demands and added expenses of raising young children on a fixed (probably lower) income. Although grandparents have played a very important role in helping to raise grandchildren, it is usually a duty of choice.

8. Menopause may not be an adaptation☺, but simply a product of the aging process itself, like decreasing acuity in the senses or metabolism slowdown. As previously mentioned, the body may be coded for menopause to occur at a certain point in the lifespan.

# 3

## *A Grieving Process?*

After much reflection, consideration, and research, there was no doubt in my mind that loss was *indeed* involved in the perimenopause process. There are actually several losses that need to be dealt with in perimenopause and ultimately menopause. A woman will confront some of these losses without choice, therefore, the loss will take place regardless (e.g. loss of the physical ability to bear children, loss/decline of the sex hormone estrogen, etc.), and other losses may or may not affect her at all (e.g. identity loss and/or role confusion, loss of/change in sociability, etc.). Some losses will be met directly as they surface, while other losses may be so subtle, that the woman may not even be aware of them. Many losses are transient and will soon pass. And, since perimenopause is so subjective and so highly individualized, one woman may experience a particular loss more intensely and for a longer duration than another woman. Furthermore, one loss is not necessarily more important or more significant than another loss. During the development phase of this book, I couldn't believe the number of losses that could in fact occur during perimenopause. And, there are probably other losses I didn't even mention.

Unfortunately, the term "loss" conjures up all sorts of bad feelings for a couple of reasons. First, there is a certain negativity attached to the word itself. And second, there is a negative connotation attached to the concept of "loss" because of its association with the dark emotional side that accompanies most loss. However, in actuality, loss *is* an important part of the life experience and one that can have very positive results. It is a universal phenomenon that we have all become familiar with in one way or another. In her book, *Necessary Losses: The Loves, Illusions, Dependencies, and Impossible Expectations That All of Us Have to Give Up in Order to Grow* (1998), Judith Viorst asserts that the many losses we experience throughout life are the norm rather than the exception and we *all* experience these losses during our lifespan. Loss is a necessary component in the course of a lifetime and is essential to our personal growth and maturation. For example, according to Judith Viorst, we lose the luxury of being dependent on our parents at some point and we must venture out on our own and become independent. We lose the grammar school years to adolescence. We lose adolescence to young adulthood. We may lose friends, yet we gain new ones. And, the list goes on. Loss is really *not* such a terrible thing as Judith Viorst asserts. In fact, it plays an integral role in our personal development.

I do want to point out that the psychological losses a woman may encounter during perimenopause are *at least* equally as important as any physical losses. Sadly though, these psychological losses have been grossly overlooked and/or completely disregarded in many professional circles. Additionally, perimenopause is *not* just a lose-lose situation. There are *many* gains that offset the losses and there are some very remarkable paradoxes that can also occur during the whole perimenopause process.

Some of the physical and psychological losses that may occur in perimenopause, and eventually menopause, include the following (*denotes a gain occurs as well and is discussed further in the "gains" section of chapter 5):

1.  Loss of the physical ability to bear children*

2.  Identity loss and/or role confusion*

3.  Loss/decline of the sex hormone estrogen

4.  Loss of the protective properties of estrogen levels that accompany the reproductive years

5.  Loss of mental consistency, i.e. irritability, mood swings (that include sudden weeping, feelings of dread, apprehension, and/or doom), anxiety, depression, feelings of helplessness, feelings of worthlessness, and/or a decrease/change in cognitive performance

6.  Loss/decline of estrogen and its relation to domestic violence

7.  Loss/decline of the sex hormone progesterone

8.  Loss of the benefits of progesterone levels that accompany the reproductive years

9.  Loss of/change in sociability*

10. Loss of/change in a caring attitude*

11. Loss of sleep/change in sleep patterns

12. Loss of/change in bladder control

13. Loss of libido (desire)/arousal/sexual functioning*

14. Loss of/change in skin tone

15. Loss of/change in hair color/quantity/texture and/or luster

16. Loss of/development of a negative self image and/or body image*

17. Loss of breast mass

18. Loss of weight control*

19. Loss of physical well being and/or a decreased quality of life*

20. Loss of confidence in decision-making ability*

21. Miscellaneous losses

Each loss presents its own distinct challenges and offers the perimenopausal woman an opportunity for psychological and spiritual growth. Let's investigate these losses further.

*Where is everyone?* I wondered. Mesmerized by the ocean surf slapping against the white sand, I carefully scanned the beach around me. There was the occasional crab sliding sideways into a burrowed hole in the sand, and the occasional seagull diving into the water for a tidbit to eat. I even spotted some activity of fish jumping in the ocean. But, except for two lifeguards sitting in their stand, the beach was virtually deserted. The ocean was just the right temperature, a mellow blue-green color, and the waves were quite small today, not rough at all. There should have been an abundance of people enjoying the beach on this most beautiful Florida day!

And, just like being the only solitary person on the entire beach that day, in spite of the beautiful ocean setting, isolation surrounded and engulfed my very soul. All the changes that I had been experiencing lately seemed to be pushing me into a world of alienation and loneliness.

Is grief and mourning involved in the perimenopause progression? This is a question that may have varied answers for different individuals. Certainly, one would not grieve for monthly cramps, discomfort, or the habitual inconveniences! However, there is genuine loss involved with perimenopause. And, as with most loss, there is mourning.

I discovered that the stages of grieving were initially associated with loss due to death and dying, as Elisabeth Kubler-Ross hypothesized in 1969. Either the terminally ill/dying individual was grieving for herself or himself in the face of death, or the individual was grieving for a loved one who was terminally ill or dying. Kubler-Ross's model hypothesized that there are certain stages an individual will confront and work through when grieving. However, since the inception of this theory, the grieving process has been greatly expanded to include *many* different aspects of loss, not only death and dying. There are numerous ways an individual might experience loss; a relationship split, a separation, a divorce, a pet's illness and/or death, loss of a home due to bankruptcy, fire, or natural disaster, empty nest syndrome, loss of a friend or family member due to relocation, divorce, illness, death, loss of a job, etc. Similarly, it appears that the losses encountered in perimenopause can propel a woman into the grieving process, without the woman even being aware of it.

According to Kubler-Ross, the grieving process is a phase (or time period) that permits a person to heal from the loss or losses suffered. It is a normal human reaction to loss that allows the individual to accept and finally adjust to the changes that have occurred. Mental adjustments and sometimes physical adjustments, such as having to move or relocate, may have to be made after experiencing a loss. There is no set manner in which one grieves and each person grieves differently and for varying lengths of time, working through the stages. One person may grieve immediately upon experiencing the loss, and yet someone else may take months or even *years* to grieve and come to grips with the loss. Some people may *never* process or even acknowledge the loss. An excellent example of a case of extremely delayed grief happened to me when my father passed on, when I was a teenage girl back in New Jersey. Even now, I can vividly remember the day my father passed. It was a chilly, windy, rainy, and very gloomy November that year, in more ways than one. He passed the day after Thanksgiving from a massive stroke. He was only sixty-two. He had been hospitalized for a week and never regained any of his faculties before passing.

*What was there to be thankful for?* I thought, as I stood shivering next to the grave site in the gusty winds and driving rain, watching him being lowered into the ground.

Although I was truly disappointed at losing the only man in the world who would have bought me the moon if he could, I really didn't grieve or even feel sadness for almost a year. The fact that I was only eighteen at the time may have had something to do with the lack of sorrow and delayed reaction. There was not one tear shed until one bitter, cold, snowy winter day, a whole calendar year afterward, as I was heading home from work in the car that he had bought for me, I broke down hysterically in tears sobbing at a red light, as the snow traveled across the windshield caught in the wipers. A chill suddenly caught me and I couldn't believe that he was really gone! In the months that followed, I wept every single day for my father most likely reacting only when the reality had hit me head-on, hitting me hard, when I finally realized that I couldn't see him, talk to him, hear him, or hug him anymore. This personal story clearly illustrates that everyone assimilates grief differently, in their own time, and on their own terms.

The remainder of this chapter documents the various losses a woman may experience during perimenopause and some losses a woman may experience at menopause. There may be other losses encountered with the passage of perimenopause that are not mentioned here, but I have attempted to capture the main ones. And, please bear in mind, there is no particular order to the listing format I have chosen; the psychological losses are interspersed with the physical losses.

First and foremost, a woman **loses her physical ability to bear children** naturally in menopause. This becomes evident to a woman in perimenopause, when there are monthly cycle alterations. If a woman has not had the opportunity to have children in her childbearing years and she would have liked to have had children, there are no more chances of producing a child once menopause has occurred. Of course, with our advanced technology today, anything is possible, but most medical data suggests that a woman *not* have children after this point. It then becomes a matter of putting the mother and the child at physical risk. Furthermore, if a woman *has* had the children she planned on having, there is still a finiteness to her fertility that exists once menopause happens. The thirty or so childbearing years that she has known and become familiar with will be lost for the remainder of her life and she now faces thirty or so non-childbearing years that will be very different in many ways. This becomes a dilemma because as humans we are mostly comfortable with the known and the familiar things in life and we are extremely *uncomfortable* with the unknown and the unfamiliar things in life. We would much rather stay in the same familiar, habitual charted territory that we have grown to live with and accept, even if that territory has disadvantages, rather than to branch out into unknown territories, even if there are benefits waiting there. We are basically creatures of habit and we like the same habits. They provide a sort of "comfort zone".

Second, due to the loss of her fertility, **identity loss and/or role confusion** may follow. If a woman's individuality and/or sole identity have been strongly defined by her childbearing capability, then she is going to have a much more difficult time accepting and managing menopause. A woman may perceive that her uniqueness as a woman is threatened once she can no longer function in a reproductive capacity. Men are capable of procreating well into old, old age. If a man suddenly became sterile and could no longer produce a child, how would he feel? Along with the other changes occurring simultaneously in the perimenopausal progression (skin changes, weight changes, etc.), a woman may feel that she is losing her femininity and/or her looks which may end up confusing her even more. She may sense that others are viewing her differently because of the many changes she is undergoing and this only compounds the intimidating nature of perimenopause.

It is damaging enough when a woman internally confronts self-doubt, but society may *also* be contributing to the identity loss and resulting insecurity a woman feels in perimenopause. My mother once told me that as you age, in this society anyway, others approach and treat you differently compared to more youthful years. I didn't believe her until I myself approached middle age. It was true! I noticed that others of all ages began treating me with somewhat less respect, with limited patience, and with decreased attentiveness. It was then that I realized that our modern culture is *definitely* designed for the young. There is no doubt about that. All you have to do is to check out at the grocery store and glance over at the magazine section. You will only occasionally see a woman on the front cover of a magazine over the age of forty-five. And, there *are* probably more middle-aged woman gracing magazine covers today than in the past, but there still remains a huge deficit in the number of middle-aged and older women appearing on magazine covers. Oprah, who recently turned fifty and looking fantastic, does appear on her magazine cover often, but then she owns the magazine!

Also, watching most reality television that has recently taken over the tube, there is rarely, *if ever*, anyone over 30 appearing on these shows (*Survivor* may be the exception). Apparently a fifty-two year old "American Idol" would be out of the question! "Do you want to marry my Dad?" was one reality show that did spotlight a middle-aged man, the Dad, as one of the main characters. But, along with him were his twenty-something year-old children who played an even greater part in the series and seemed to have been given much more air time than their middle-aged Dad. This is consistent with the observation that our modern society, in general, imposes a *powerful* sense of pressure on individuals, especially women, to maintain a youthful appearance. And, these societal demands in turn, add unnecessary stress to the aging woman. She may question her maturation and attractiveness and feel less sexually desirable in a culture where youth rules.

As a final thought concerning **identity loss and/or role confusion**, if you think about it, sexuality actually consists of many other elements above and beyond the biological reproductive component. Because a woman can no longer physically create offspring does *not* decrease or eliminate her sexuality or sensuality! There is the sensual nature to humans that transcends the physical procreation function, therefore, there is human intimacy, love, and pleasure that also comprises sexuality/sensuality. And, these features of human sexuality continue on until one passes from this earth.

Third, there is a **loss of the sex hormone estrogen** in perimenopause. Estrogen is actually a *group* or *family* of hormones, not just one distinct hormone.[30] There are three main components in the estrogen family as follows: (1) Estradiol is the primary estrogen produced in the ovaries. After menopause, this estrogen drops. (2) Estrone is formed from estradiol, a weak estrogen that is the most abundant estrogen found in the body after menopause. And, (3) Estriol is produced in large amounts during pregnancy. It is a breakdown product of estradiol. And, it may have anti-cancer effects.[31]

Estrogen has *three hundred* identified functions in the body making it an *extremely* important hormone. Besides being fundamental in the reproductive process and being responsible for uterus and breast development in the female, estrogen has *many* other beneficial effects on the body, both physical and psychological. Some of the other benefits of estrogen are:

1.   Estrogen stimulates the production of the neurotransmitter, serotonin, which plays a role in the brain as a mood elevator. Estrogen also stimulates the production of the neurotransmitter, acetylcholine, which is essential for memory.[32] Both of these neurotransmitters are depleted in Alzheimer's patients.

2.   Estrogen is believed to activate the temporary growth of nerve pathways in the memory section of the brain.

3.   The relationship between estrogen and the brain chemical serotonin plays an important role in restful sleep.

4.   Estrogen exerts its power on blood vessels by smoothing, relaxing, and opening them, which may increase blood flow to the brain.

5.   Estrogen has protective properties on the heart by increasing HDL, the good cholesterol, and decreasing LDL, the harmful cholesterol.

6.  Estrogen assists in building healthy bones and prevents bone break-down. It may play a role in the existence of osteoclasts (cells responsible in bone breakdown). It also plays a role in sustaining levels of Vitamin D, a nutrient found to protect bones.

7.  Estrogen maintains the body's thermostat.

8.  Estrogen appears to offer protection against glaucoma, macular degeneration, and cataracts.

9.  Estrogen is an antioxidant.

There are many, many more functions that estrogen plays a role in, too many to list here. But, you get the picture. It is quite apparent, from the above mentioned items, that estrogen exerts powerful, positive, protective, and supportive properties on a woman's physical and mental health and well being. It is not surprising then that estrogen loss is probably *the* major contributing factor to perimenopausal signs that a woman may develop during perimenopause.

So…fourth, it follows that with the loss of estrogen production in perimenopause, a woman **loses the protective properties that accompany higher estrogen levels found in the reproductive years**. Estrogen production will eventually decline to about one-third of what it was in a woman's childbearing years. And, without the beneficial qualities that estrogen offers, there can be susceptibility to problems. For instance, in the **physical realm** during perimenopause, bone mass begins to decline from estrogen loss, and a woman can lose from 0.5% to 6% of her bone mass per year, resulting in vulnerability to **osteoporosis**, which is the loss of bone density. In osteoporosis, the bone becomes weaker than a normal bone and can fracture easier. It is astounding how many women are affected by osteoporosis! In fact, eight million of the ten million people in the U.S. who have osteoporosis are women.[33] Men can get osteoporosis too—approximately two million American men have osteoporosis.[34] And…it is estimated that approximately 34 million *more* Americans may have **low bone density**.[35] But, women are at a higher risk than men of getting osteoporosis because women's bones commonly tend to be smaller than men's bones according to The National Osteoporosis Foundation.

It should be mentioned that even though estrogen does play an important role in the maintenance of bone health, there are other risk factors that also place a woman at higher risk of getting osteoporosis. For example, osteoporosis can happen in a woman who has had her ovaries surgically removed, or in a woman who experiences early menopause.[36] A small or thin body frame, being Caucasian or

Asian, inadequate calcium in the diet, a family history, a smoking history, an alcohol history, or even physical inactivity can put a woman at greater risk of getting osteoporosis.[37]

Another physical sign that may arise during perimenopause are **hot flashes**. Due to estrogen production declines and its connection to the hypothalamus, the body's internal thermostat is affected, hence hot flashes occur (the hypothalamus detects and responds to lower estrogen levels by changing the body's temperature).[38] A **hot flash** is the sensation of a sudden rush of heat in the neck, face, and/or other areas of the body that can last from a few seconds to many minutes.[39] They come and they go. A woman may suddenly feel hot and then feel cold. This is one of the most commonly occurring perimenopausal signs—85% of American perimenopausal women experience hot flashes and 10% of women will still experience them up to ten years later.[40]

Then, there are those similar (and equally as irritating) **night sweats** that are also caused by estrogen fluctuations during perimenopause. I started experiencing these night sweats near the end of my 45th year. It was initially difficult to pinpoint what was happening to me since I live in Florida, and it is *always* hot here. Sometimes during the night, I would be awakened by an extreme feeling of warmth all over; it felt as if my whole body was burning up. It was similar to a fever—like my body was on fire, except that I never really was one to sweat, so I just felt awfully hot.

I would get up and check out the air conditioning system, which seemed to run almost non-stop especially during the summer months. It was the same temperature that it was every other night. There didn't seem to be anything wrong with the A/C system.

Then, I would make my way to my son's room on the other side of the house, and if he was still awake, I would question him, "Are you hot in here?"

"No." He would answer.

Then I knew it was me.

My sister-in-law expressed this feeling of night sweats well. "I feel like my body is 200°!"

**Perimenopausal insomnia** may also occur because the connection between estrogen and the neurotransmitter serotonin changes with falling estrogen levels. A hot flash or night sweats may also interfere with a good night's sleep. And, we all know that night after sleepless night can take its toll on our physical health as well as our psychological wellness.

Additionally, in post menopause, **heart disease** rates rise among women, due to a loss of estrogen and its protective influence on the cardiovascular system. Blood pressure, blood fats, cholesterol, and blood glucose [41] can all be affected.

These are only a *few* of the problems that can arise when estrogen levels decline during perimenopause and overall physical health is affected. Be advised that the potential problems mentioned here are not all inclusive due to the *numerous* protective properties estrogen has on the body. And, you will find that I have listed other estrogen related losses that deserve their own mention in the remainder of this chapter.

One of the very first signs of perimenopause that *I* noticed in myself was connected to this estrogen loss. Almost every single one of my **joints** began to ache! I experienced arthralgia☺ some days very intensely. My ankles, knees, elbows, wrists, and even my fingers were all affected (the shoulders and hips were spared for the time being). The initial aches started in my elbows of all places. One day, I woke up to aching elbows. Not just one elbow, but both elbows. They weren't inflamed or tender to the touch and they seemed to work okay. But, upon movement they were stiff and sore.

*What is going on?* I contemplated, upon waking. I silently lay awake mentally covering a myriad of activities from the previous day that could have caused hurting elbows.

*Did I bang them on something? Did I lean on them? Did I misuse them in some way that I was unaware of?* And then, every other possible reason for elbow pain popped into my mind. *Was it the rainy weather? Was I lacking something in my diet? Was I just getting older and these discomforts were merely signs of the aging process? Was it arthritis? Would the aching go away? Wasn't this something that only happened to very old people?* I was only forty-five, hardly considered old by present day standards. *Didn't this just affect people with arthritis? Why was I having all this joint pain and stiffness?*

The aching lasted a day or so and then it would disappear altogether for a few days to a few weeks. The general nature of the pain was ambiguous and unpredictable, and more of a nuisance than anything else. It came and went.

Subsequently, my knees started bothering me. Once again, not one knee, but both knees ached. And, as with most joint pain, it bothered me more upon waking in the morning. I was on a walking regimen at the time that included three miles three to four times a week. So…of course, I attributed any aches and pains to the exercise. It was a *wonderful* excuse to stop exercising, which I disliked anyway. However, to my surprise, once I discontinued the walking routine, the joint pain continued to flare up in both knees.

Strangely enough, I didn't seem to have one elbow and one knee hurting at the same time, but the pain surfaced as an elbow and an elbow, a knee and a knee, an ankle and an ankle. The discomfort usually appeared bilaterally when it presented—maybe because I was focused on that one particular joint when it hurt? And at other times, my fingers would become very stiff and it would be a struggle to straighten out or extend all of my fingers. Prior to conducting any research on perimenopause, I was *totally* unaware of the cause for all of these joint discomforts. Who would ordinarily blame intermittent joint aches on internal hormone levels? Somehow, they just didn't seem to go together! But…sure enough, to my downright amazement, estrogen declines were *absolutely* responsible for joint stiffness and aching.

As a final point on the loss of the protective properties of estrogen during perimenopause, there are **psychological signs** that may also appear as a result of estrogen declines. Mood swings, irritability, anxiety, depression, and cognitive changes, to mention a few, may surface during perimenopause. These are discussed in detail in the next loss.

In the fifth loss, there may be a **loss of mental consistency, i.e. irritability, mood swings (that includes sudden weeping, feelings of dread, apprehension, and/or doom), anxiety, depression, feelings of helplessness, feelings of worthlessness,[42] and/or a decrease/change in cognitive performance**. There are three distinct theories that have offered some explanation for mental inconsistency during perimenopause.[43] The **first theory** concentrates on "**Estrogen Declines**".[44] As I mentioned previously, mental functioning is rather dependent on circulating hormone levels and their interaction on the central nervous system (CNS). Estrogen receptors appear in large numbers in the brain's limbic area (memory and emotional behavior), and estrogen also assists in nerve growth, nerve repair, and general neural activity. With a decline in estrogen levels during perimenopause, attention, concentration, verbal and spatial memory, and long and short term memory are some of the cognitive functions that may be affected. Irritability, mood swings, anxiousness, depression, feelings of helplessness and/or feelings of worthlessness may also surface during perimenopause that, according to this first theory, could be due to estrogen loss.

It has been speculated in the **second theory** that mental inconsistency during perimenopause may occur because of a "**Domino Effect**".[45] Therefore, any physical changes that occur during perimenopause such as sleepless nights, hot flashes, night sweats, vaginal dryness, etc. may lead to mental changes such as fatigue, irritability, loss of libido, etc. by creating a domino effect. An alteration in cognitive performance such as memory disruption, for example, could be due to a lack of sleep. Or, fatigue could result in increased anxiety, impatience, or other altered behaviors.

The **third theory** attempting to explain mental inconsistencies during perimenopause is called the "**Stage of Life**" theory.[46] This theory asserts that the external life events and other peripheral stresses a woman may be experiencing during perimenopause are actually to blame for mental inconsistencies and not the perimenopause process itself. Significant life events such as an empty nest, aging or ill family members, career pressures/demands/changes, financial pressures/demands/changes, spouse or partner issues, etc. are believed to affect a woman's moods and behaviors.

Expounding on the three above mentioned theories, it is my belief that instead of putting any one particular theory above another, it is more likely that a *combination* of the three theories plays a role in causing mental inconsistencies during perimenopause. I can clearly see how *each* of these theories affected my own behavior to a certain degree. For example, the "**Stage of Life**" theory could explain why my moods were affected more when external events transpired in my life and stress levels increased, i.e. when I lost my job and had financial worries. Similarly, the "**Estrogen**" theory could explain why my moods and behavior were affected more at other times, like when I was experiencing joint aches, headaches, etc.

I should mention that many different studies have been done involving diminishing levels of hormones in perimenopause (and menopause) and changes in mental performance. There are opposing findings and assertions on the topic. Some results from these analyses indicate that there *are* mental declines along with hormonal declines. And, other studies resulted in *no* correlation whatsoever between any mental declines and hormonal declines. For purposes of this book, I will *support* the belief that decreasing hormone levels do *indeed* affect mental functioning, since I have personally experienced some cognitive variances, depression, mood swings, irritability, and anxiety during perimenopause. And, because of the nature and timing of onset, I would have to attribute these many psychological changes to hormonal declines.

Below, I have documented some of the psychological changes prompted by perimenopause that I noticed in my own mental functioning and emotionality. These mental changes include mental intrusions/exclusions, intense and sudden emotion, irritability, anxiety, forgetfulness, depression, etc.—many mental inconsistencies that other women may also experience during perimenopause.

## Irritability/Short fuse:

A loss of patience was slowly creeping into my daily life and I noticed a significant difference in my day-to-day attitude. As my son approached adolescence, *I* was approaching perimenopause. What an explosive combination to be living under one roof at the *same* time! It was quite interesting to say the least. Referring to my son's erratic and self-absorbed emotional adolescent behavior as "hormonal", here I was experiencing the same "hormonal" behavior—unpredictable, irritable, introspective, and sometimes *so* self-regarding. I recognized that many events and/or situations that I had dealt with so easily on a daily basis prior to this perimenopausal state, were now becoming a problem. A *big* problem. In my mind's eye, my perception of certain situations was becoming intensely exaggerated in importance and scope. For example, prior to perimenopause, if my son would ask me for the fifth time if a friend could come over, I would typically continue answering him in a calm voice. "We'll see," I would respond until I could reach a definitive decision. Now though, I found myself responding with an emphatic and forceful "No!" by the second time he asked me the same thing. His unwavering persistence really started to irritate me these days when it never had before. In fact, I always admired his perseverance and determination in pursuing what he wanted because I knew that someday, this characteristic would be useful for him.

Other drivers on the road *really* started aggravating me too with their poor driving habits and slow reaction times. If another driver suddenly pulled in front of me without warning, causing me to stop abruptly, my heart would start to race, and I would have a few choice words for that driver. I even caught myself expressing these obscenities out loud a few times! Or, if someone in front of me was driving 20 MPH slower than the designated speed limit (remember I live in Florida), I would have a few more descriptive words for *that* driver. Ordinarily, I would just pass the slowpoke and forget about it, but nowadays things like this really bothered me.

"Please press 2 if you wish to speak with a customer service representative," the prerecorded message stated. One day, while on the telephone with my insurance company, after being directed to the *fifth* separate prerecorded message for what seemed like hours, I had a few *more* choice words for the robotic and humanless interaction that the world was subjected to! As I sat impatiently waiting for the sixth prerecorded message, I noticed a definite pattern emerging in my behavior, namely insignificant minor daily irritations were eliciting *major* reactions from me, whereas before they wouldn't even raise an eyebrow.

It seemed quite obvious to me that in my younger years, I was much more patient and tolerant of every day situations. It was strange, because I had always thought that together with age came patience, tolerance, and fortitude. But, contrary to those prior beliefs, instead of gaining the characteristics that could help me cope with the complexities of life, these qualities were vanishing lately. I was becoming irritable, short-tempered, and intolerant of people and situations in general.

*Hopefully, this was only a temporary state.* I considered.

## Intense/Sudden emotion (sadness, weeping):

Not only was my fuse short, but I would become *very* emotional *very* quickly. I might be watching Oprah, Montel, or the news and suddenly my eyes would start tearing up if a particular topic touched me. Or, if I started thinking about my father, who passed on when I was 18, my eyes would suddenly well up. Hadn't I processed this loss years ago? This sudden, intense emotion was *very* different behavior for me as I was usually in total control of my emotions at all times. But lately, I felt like I was completely *losing* control of my emotions. And, I didn't like it.

In the past, I found that auditory imagery (a mental image that is similar to an auditory perception)[47] was a fantastic coping strategy that helped relieve increased anxiety levels that I was experiencing. So...I tried applying this same coping strategy to the sudden and sometimes intense emotional situations in perimenopause and to my surprise it worked! If I was having a "perimenopausal moment", i.e. feeling blue, weeping, etc. I would quickly try to think of a certain song to counteract the intense emotion that I was experiencing.

I first began using this mental imagery a few years back, on the day that I defended my thesis. I was driving to my college to appear before three professors to defend my thesis which represented a year's worth of research and statistics that I had worked on. It was about a 25 minute drive north leaving me *plenty* of time to work myself up into a panicked state. I was *so* nervous—I didn't know *how* I was going to maintain my composure during the hour long presentation. As my mind drifted off deeper into anxiousness, a song suddenly appeared on the car radio that surprisingly snapped me out of my anxiety-ridden state in an instant. It was an older song by Phil Collins, *Another Day in Paradise*, that spoke of a woman who was pretty much down on her luck—a bag lady who had no real place to call home. The chorus started as I listened, "Oh think twice, it's just another day for you and me in paradise." It was actually a very sad song, but interestingly enough, at this very moment in time, it made *me* begin to feel better and to gain some confidence in myself.

*How many poor people are living in this country?* I thought to myself.

*On second thought, how many poor, underprivileged people are living in this world who would die to have a college education, and who would die to be driving to their college in their car to defend their thesis.* This particular thought quickly relieved the intense anxiety that I had been experiencing about defending my thesis. And, I suddenly considered myself to be a very lucky girl—living in a country where, not only as a person, but as a woman, I could pursue an education, and where people (my professors) really wanted me to succeed. The anxious nature of the drive was immensely decreased after listening to that song, and I continued to my thesis defense appointment in a much more positive frame of mind, focusing on the positive aspects of the experience. I have used that particular song *many, many* times since, to successfully reduce any anxiety that I might be experiencing. And most recently, this particular song had succeeded in reducing the intense *emotions* that I was currently experiencing during this perimenopausal state.

Thank God for music.

## Depression:

Lately, I had been feeling very down in the dumps. But, there were *so* many *other* external circumstances occurring at the same time as perimenopause that it would be too difficult to separate out the exact cause of the blues. My gloomy spirits could easily have been the outcome of any *one* of a number of other stressful events that were also happening in my life. I found myself forgetting things all the time too—forgetting certain words, forgetting past events, forgetting things at the store, forgetting what I just said! During my research, I discovered that forgetfulness may not only be a result of hormonal declines, but it may actually be triggered by depression. Depression can affect memory (or lack of it) by causing trouble in concentration and by causing distractibility leading to retention problems.[48] Also, the motivation and driving forces that keep us going on a daily basis decline to much lower levels in depression making memory retrieval problematic.[49]

Even though perimenopause seemed a likely cause of my depression, there is conflicting evidence linking depression to perimenopause and to menopause. Some studies found that up to 40% of menopausal women suffered some depression during this time. And, statistics from some menopause clinics revealed that depression *was* a frequent complaint from women who were seeking medical advice during perimenopause.[50] An increased rate of transitory depression was found in women who faced a *lengthy* perimenopause with negative signs.[51] A limited or lack of a social support network seemed to contribute to feelings of depression and a bad intimate relationship was also found to be responsible for feelings of depression during perimenopause.[52]

According to a report in the Archives of General Psychiatry, life-long or continued depression and financial hardships may actually lead to an early menopause.[53] Consistent with that finding, according to the National Women's Health Information Center, some studies found that women with a history of depression *did* enter menopause earlier than those women experiencing no depression. And, women who were on antidepressant medications entered perimenopause even sooner.[54]

However, The Pittsburgh findings, which were supported by a New England Research Institute study, found that menopausal depression appeared no more frequently than in the general population; 10% of menopausal women were occasionally depressed and 5% were persistently depressed, which is consistent with depression in the general population. This study also indicated that those women most at risk of depression were surgically induced menopausal women whose depression rate was almost *double* that of naturally menopausal women.[55]

Feelings of helplessness and/or feelings of worthlessness may also surface in depression. These feelings can be fleeting or they can continue throughout the perimenopause phase. However often or intense they actually do occur, these feelings *can* be overwhelming for the perimenopausal woman.[56]

## Anxiety/Mood swings/disorders:

Also accompanying perimenopause was a steady increase in my anxiety levels. I had always been a somewhat anxious person by nature, but now my nerves were really shot. Lately the anxiety would overwhelm me. My heart would race from time-to-time and I would experience heart palpitations. This could also happen from estrogen level fluctuations, but it seemed to occur mostly when I found myself in an anxiety-provoking situation. I discovered that perimenopause could indeed exacerbate prior mood disorders—disorders of emotion and affect. Mood disorders could recur as described in the "vulnerability theory"* therefore the mood disorder could surface again or become more noticeable during the menopausal transition. For that very reason, this current hormonal state reintroduced high anxiety levels that I had experienced before perimenopause.

Additionally, I discovered that not only can prior mood disorders surface during perimenopause, but new onset mood disorders can also appear during this transition.

**\*The Vulnerability Theory** asserts that if a woman had a mood disorder *before* the menopausal transition, then she may be at an increased risk of that same mood disorder *during* the menopause transition.57

## Foggy Thinking, Fuzzy Thinking, or Fuzzy Head:

In addition to the recent forgetfulness I was experiencing "foggy thinking", "fuzzy thinking", or "fuzzy head" as it is sometimes referred to, sometimes my mind just felt like it was in a "fog". Any level-headedness I thought I possessed went right out the window with the onset of perimenopause! There are opposing findings and assertions (once again) on the exact cause of foggy thinking, fuzzy thinking, or fuzzy head during perimenopause that is not due to depression. Some researchers believe that estrogen fluctuations or declines *do* play a role in memory performance and yet other researchers assert that there is *no* connection between estrogen and memory performance in perimenopause.[58] Whatever the cause, fuzzy head does seem to go away after the menopausal transition.[59]

I do want to point out here that during the course of all my research for this book, there seemed to be opposing findings on just about *everything*! I realized that what one researcher/group/individual believed/found/reported was not necessarily what another researcher/group/individual believed/found/reported. And, of course, the sample population of any study must always be considered. I realized that maybe the real answer actually included a little bit of both sides. A woman would be wise to sift through the information and take into account her own beliefs/feelings/findings/signs and come to her own conclusions.

As a final thought on the fifth loss of mental consistency, remember that besides affecting a woman's physical health, perimenopause has the power to reach into *every* aspect of her psychological being too, i.e. her overall behavior, her moods, her patience/tolerance levels, her thought processes, her memory, her self esteem, etc. And, the way a woman feels about herself, carries herself, and takes care of herself during this time is undeniably related to the entire perimenopause process.

In the sixth loss, it has been asserted that **estrogen loss during perimenopause may actually be associated with the amount of domestic violence\* a woman experiences** for a couple of reasons:

\*The Centers for Disease Control and Prevention (CDC) defines **domestic violence** as: intimate partner violence. An intimate partner may be a dating partner, a domestic partner, a spouse, or a partner from a prior intimate relationship.[60]

(1) **She may be the aggressor**. Interestingly, even though the rate of domestic violence (male-on-female violence) generally decreases with age, there is evidence suggesting that the **percentage and severity of domestic violence that is committed by women (female-on-male violence)** *increases* **with age!**[61] The current research is fairly sparse, but it *has* been speculated that the **estrogen declines/ fluctuations in perimenopause** may be to blame. One survey (Stets and Straus) found that *two thirds* of the domestic violence in couples living together aged 45 and up, was female violence directed toward the male partner.[62] And, other extreme violence by women peaked between the ages of 35–44, exactly when estrogen levels start the decline.[63] As previously stated, a woman's patience levels during perimenopause can be lowered and the fuse shortened during this time of life. And, when a woman is experiencing perimenopause at the same time she is (1) being challenged with other significant life events, (2) dealing with her own set of perimenopausal issues, (3) being confronted with multiple demands, i.e. working, taking care of a home and children, going to school, caring for/worrying about an elderly/ill parent, etc., (4) experiencing financial problems, (5) in a poor relationship, (6) dealing with a troubled teen or another problem child, (7) dealing with a myriad of other problems, is this staggering percentage of female perpetrated violence really that surprising?

(2) **She may provoke the aggression**. A perimenopausal woman may also inadvertently end up provoking unwanted responses or even domestic violence from a partner in a torrent of fluctuating hormones. A partner may be totally unprepared and/or uninformed on how to deal with the woman's perimenopausal experience, resulting in frustration, arguments, and worse yet domestic violence.

And lastly, as a woman matures beyond middle age, she may be at a higher risk of domestic violence (male directed toward female violence) if her partner was abusive in the past or the relationship was strained when they were younger.[64]

Appearing seventh on the list of losses, there is a **decline in progesterone levels** being produced in the ovaries (smaller amounts are produced in the adrenal glands). Actually, progesterone is almost *absent* in the menopausal woman.[65] Progesterone is another sex hormone that is extremely important for a healthy body inside and out. During the reproductive process it is responsible for stimulating the lining of the uterus where the baby develops, assists the breasts in milk production, and helps maintain the pregnancy. It has many other functions including contributing to nerve cells, brain cells, the thyroid gland, and muscles as well as assisting with energy and fat metabolism.[66] Some of the functions of progesterone are:

1. Progesterone normalizes blood clotting.

2. Progesterone assists in maintaining oxygen levels in the cells.

3. Progesterone normalizes zinc and copper levels, thereby decreasing moodiness.

4. Progesterone is a natural antidepressant.

5. Progesterone works with the neurotransmitter, GABA, in promoting restful sleep.

6. Progesterone helps the body use fat for energy.

So…it follows that in the eighth loss as a result of declining progesterone levels, there is a **loss of the benefits of the hormone progesterone**. With the dramatic reduction of this hormone in perimenopause, a woman will lose the protective advantages it offers. There will be susceptibility to lowered energy levels, moodiness, sleep disturbances, aching joints, and the list goes on.

Ninth, relating to the irritability, the mood swings, the depression, and the anxiety in perimenopause, there may be a pronounced **loss of sociability**. Not only was my diminishing patience level affecting interpersonal relationships, but increasing anxiety levels were interfering with casual outside sociable interaction as well. Maybe this simply comes with the aging process, but I was cutting people out of *my* life left and right! This was something that I had *never* done before and it made me very uncomfortable, yet in the end I was relieved and actually felt liberated. I found myself conducting a sort of **personal inventory** with the people around me at this mid-point in my life. When I mentioned this inventory process to some of my closer friends and contemporaries, they too stated that they were conducting their own personal life inventories! They admitted to weeding through a multitude of friendships eliminating the stale, mentally draining, and unhealthy relationships. I began to measure the value of every single person in my life. And, to my naïve surprise, I realized that *many* of the people in my life were not as important as I had once believed. There was no give and take going on. It was all give. Mainly, I felt like I was the one doing all of the giving. Many of these so called "friends" would take hour after hour of my time unburdening their problems and life difficulties on me only to abandon me when I needed *their* emotional support the most.

*Who hadn't suffered some hard times in this world?* I thought. I myself had suffered misfortunes. But for me, friendship represented a two-way street involving *mutual* communication.

Time after time, hour after hour was spent listening and giving advice to friends and acquaintances, until I finally realized that when *I* needed to discuss my *own* problems, I got about 3 minutes out of a 2 hour conversation! The other 117 minutes was spent discussing their problems. As these so-called "friends" discussed their own trials and tribulations, it eventually became very obvious to me that they really didn't care about me at all. They simply needed some counseling, which I was always willing to give. My anxiety levels were on the rise too, probably from all of the free counseling that I was giving and from becoming overly involved in their problems and excessively drawn into their predicaments. Consequently, I decided to cut all of the dead wood from my life during this perimenopause phase.

Another element of my socializing that was influenced by perimenopause was something unusual—something, I was sure, that many people had learned in high school or even earlier. And, here *I* was in middle adulthood, just learning this most valuable life lesson. This particular aspect of socializing had to do with mentally considering others' motives and agendas. I had always taken people at face value; in other words, whatever they told me, I believed. I was a very naïve person in that respect. I truly thought that people were basically good-hearted and honest. But, after a couple of inconsistencies surfaced with a few co-workers (toward the end of my employment), I was beginning to have my doubts about their motives. And after speaking with my analyst, it became crystal clear to me that *totally* trusting and believing *everything* everyone said was not in my best interest, especially in the workplace.

"You'll have to learn to practice **healthy skepticism**," he would say. A term he used meaning: use cautious awareness when interacting with others. With "healthy skepticism", I needed to modify my psyche so that it resembled a computer that filtered out junk mail—listen to what people were telling me and discard what I thought or felt to be junk, therefore, not taking every word they spoke as the gospel truth.

With help from my analyst, I discovered that people learned things when they were ready to learn them. I realized that many lessons were actually *always* there waiting to be learned, but were learned only when the individual was ready to learn them. Some people did grasp this lesson of "healthy skepticism" very early on, but until I had been exposed to the insincerities and misrepresentations of others, and acknowledged them, only *then* did I get the message and learn the real meaning. The very same lesson that some people were fortunate enough to have learned in high school or even earlier in life, I was learning in the middle of my life in perimenopause!

At this point, I should mention that with *all* of the losses that I was experiencing in my own personal perimenopause, there was also *tremendous* psychological and spiritual growth that was occurring at the same time. I was learning things that I was surprised to be learning so late in life, while also gaining valuable insight into life. Each loss became an opportunity for introspection and sometimes modification in my current behavior. For instance, now armed with "healthy skepticism" in my back pocket, I would *never* again view another person who entered my life without pulling it out of my pocket and using it. It was a *fantastic* tool for aiding in a true perception of others.

The final component in a loss of sociability during perimenopause is the fact that the perimenopausal woman may become *so* **temperamental** that no one really wants to be around her! The mood swings and volatility may result in chasing others away, affecting her social life *enormously*. This may even be a time when a relationship split/separation/divorce occurs, especially if the two have been unhappy with the relationship but remained together for reasons other than they really liked each other. And, with a relationship split/separation/divorce, may come a loss of family and friends, resulting in the loss of a stable social network. Unfortunately, losing this support network may happen at the very time the perimenopausal woman needs a support system the most. Lastly, not only are some break-ups due to a perimenopausal woman's mood swings and short fuse, but as I mentioned earlier, she may also be conducting a sort of life audit and the choice for a relationship split/separation/divorce becomes hers.

Appearing tenth on the list of losses during perimenopause, which is also closely related to a loss in mental consistency, is the **loss of a caring attitude**. By this, I don't mean that the woman consciously harms or wishes harm on others, but there is a blasé attitude that develops during perimenopause that may have never existed before. This particular loss may develop in the perimenopausal woman without her having any awareness of it, until suddenly, one day she just wakes up and doesn't care about the same things any more (note: this is also consistent with a priority assessment and/or a priority shift further discussed in the next chapter). That is *exactly* how an overall change in attitude slithered into my perimenopausal days. One day, I simply didn't seem to care about the same things I used to care about. As stated above in the ninth loss, cutting people out of my life bothered me at first, but then I really didn't care anymore. In my younger years, I would have felt absolutely terrible about ignoring someone or not responding to them, but now I felt that if people weren't good in my life, they shouldn't be a part of it.

I truly believe that this "I don't care" attitude really helped me become much more comfortable and content with myself. It was as if I was settling into a nice big chair, wrapped in a warm blanket, in front of a crackling fire. It was sort of ironic because as irritable as I could become, I was actually settling into myself. I was becoming seasoned with life. I figured my life was already half over, and I didn't want to waste any more time on nonsense. The people who didn't really care about me and the superfluous things in this life (especially if you didn't own the material things outright and had to work hard to make payments on them) were energy consumers and I didn't want to squander any more of my precious energy on wasteful things.

I also didn't care any more what the forties looked like on me. Recognizing in the mirror one morning that the twenties and the thirties had marched on and the forties were here to stay, I was just happy to be alive and I didn't care any more about the twenties and the thirties or the way I looked in them! I wanted to be the best that I could be every day here in my forties. The simple things in life seemed to matter to me nowadays, not a wrinkle on my face, not a few extra pounds, not all the materialistic, plastic paraphernalia, or all the trappings of this physical life. In actuality, I was becoming lower maintenance than I had *ever* been before, less materialistic, and much more spiritual. I also started taking inventory in my house with my personal belongings. The things I didn't care about any more were given to Goodwill or thrown out if they were beyond use. This "I don't care" attitude, actually turned out to be an extremely positive catalyst for a spring cleaning or personal inventory in the middle of my life (or should I say fall cleaning, entering the winter of my life).

In the eleventh loss, there may be a **loss of sleep** during perimenopause. Sleep is *extremely* important for healthy daily functioning physically and mentally and it should not be overlooked or underestimated as it so often is. Normal sleep patterns are *frequently* altered with declining estrogen levels in perimenopause, usually resulting in less sleep and/or disruptive sleep. Sleep problems may also arise because of hot flashes and/or night sweats that can occur throughout the night. And, urinary frequency and/or incontinence may require repeated bathroom trips during the night disrupting sleep as well. This particular inconvenience is caused by a loss of tissue tone due to (once again) decreased estrogen levels. Even though I had always heard to hydrate throughout the day and evening, I found that withholding large amounts of liquids after 7 p.m. helped me to have a more restful night's sleep. Most of the time, I would only take small amounts of water after this time. For me, a good night's sleep was *much* more important than hydrating in the evening and then spending the rest of the night making numerous trips to the bathroom. Additionally, making sure there was a trip to the bathroom *immediately* before going to bed every night helped me avoid waking up throughout the night.

Furthermore, persistent disruptions in normal sleep patterns can have a negative effect on the body. Sleep deprivation can result in decreased energy levels, decreased work performance, and difficulties in concentrating. It can also increase the risk of auto accidents (fall asleep accidents) and can intensify any pain or discomfort a perimenopausal woman may be experiencing.[67] Sleep disruptions can also affect a woman's cognitive functioning by contributing to memory loss, as sleep has been associated with reinforcing memories and in processing complex emotions. Sleep deprivation can also affect other functions many of us don't even think about. For instance, loss of sleep can affect metabolism and *increase* hunger. A loss of sleep has been blamed for increased blood pressure and it can create a much shorter fuse in the perimenopausal woman leaving her at risk for depression and other mood disorders.

The twelfth loss in perimenopause may involve a **change in bladder control**. Estrogen assists in maintaining the lining of the bladder and urethra and it also assists in keeping the pelvic muscles strong. With the estrogen declines in perimenopause, there can be a weakening of the pelvic muscles that are responsible for bladder control. And, these changes may result in leaking of urine, especially while coughing or sneezing (stress incontinence) or there may be a sense of urgency (urge incontinence).

The next loss and perhaps the source of *many* disagreements with a partner, there may be a **loss of libido (desire), arousal, and/or sexual functioning** with the onset of perimenopause. There are several components involved in sexual functioning that can all be affected in perimenopause.[68] They include, for example, desire, arousal, motivation, satisfaction, pleasure (giving and receiving), there are those fantasies, and there is the orgasm itself.[69] Most of these sexual elements are influenced to some degree by the hormonal declines in perimenopause.[70] The **physiological explanations** include the following: (1) The fact that the ovaries are no longer producing testosterone, the sex hormone responsible for a sex drive in both men and women. The adrenal glands will produce a small amount of testosterone, but not in the same quantities that the ovaries once produced. (2) Estrogen and androgens are also involved in sexual functioning.[71] And, with a diminishing supply of estrogen in perimenopause, the vagina may become thinner, lack lubrication, and/or lack elasticity making intercourse uncomfortable and/or painful for the perimenopausal woman. (3) Decreasing estrogen levels play a negative role in nerve impulses during sex as well, resulting in less sensitivity.[72] And, (4) declining estrogen levels also play a role in lessening the arousal response, due to decreased blood flow to sexually sensitive areas.[73] Some women will regain the same sexual interest they experienced in earlier years once things settle down. However, some women will not ever have the same sexual interest. In fact, after menopause, approximately a third of women will experience a decreased sex drive.[74]

**Psychological factors** that can influence a woman's sexual outlook and sexual drive during perimenopause include the following: (1) Other life pressures the perimenopausal woman may be experiencing at this point in life may be overwhelming for her. (2) Societal norms/expectations/influences about aging can be a powerful force on a woman's sexuality. (3) A woman's *own* overall attitude/anxieties/fears toward aging can greatly affect her sexuality.[75] (4) Sex may once have been a priority that now takes a back seat to other things, i.e. a priority shift. And, (5) a negative body image can considerably affect a woman's sex drive/arousal/functioning. This will be discussed a little later in this chapter.

Another sexual problem that may arise during perimenopause is **sexual incompatibility**. A couple may have been sexually compatible during most of their relationship, only to find that during the menopausal transition, the perimenopausal woman is not as interested in sex as she once was. This can be a *real* dilemma in that the sexual nature of the relationship has already been clearly defined. And, with the onset of perimenopause that may result in a lowered sexual interest, there is now an alteration in prior sexual expectations and routines that must be redefined. Or, the perimenopausal woman may begin to experience discomfort or difficulty in the sex act itself resulting in a decreased interest in sex which can also create a rift in the sexual relationship.

Now that the obvious physiological and psychological reasons for a waning libido, arousal, and sexual functioning in perimenopause have been considered, there are other **more analytical theories** that deserve mention. They are as follows:

1. This is simply nature's way of dealing with the fact that a menopausal woman is no longer able to bear children. If procreating is the main function of the sex act, as some cultures and religions believe, then why would a woman want or need to engage in sex if she can no longer create offspring?

2.  Following the above reason, after investing time and effort into finding a suitable father for her offspring during the childbearing years, her family is most likely established and/or ready to leave home. Why would any more investment in this process, i.e. flirting, courtship, etc. be necessary?

3.  A significant other/husband is probably aging right along with the perimenopausal woman (unless she has opted for a younger man). Men go through similar changes as women that accompany aging, i.e. skin differences, thinning hair, weight gain, etc. Maybe he no longer turns the perimenopausal woman on?

4.  The perimenopausal woman may have been in a poor relationship/marriage for years and perimenopause, with all of its challenges, only contributes to distancing the couple even further.

5.  Finally, some women will *consciously* choose to become less sexually active at the time of menopause. One Swedish study found that some women used menopause as an excuse to put an end to sex after years of disinterest.[76]

Appearing fourteenth on the list of losses during perimenopause is a **loss of or a change in skin tone.**

*Who is this person?* I questioned myself, applying my make-up one morning. *Do I know this person?* Lately, the person staring back at me in the mirror looked like somebody I didn't know. There were distinct signs of aging appearing as small lines distributed around my face, mostly around my eyes (crow's feet), and some lines around my mouth. Oh my God! I suddenly realized one morning *who* the reflection in the mirror resembled. It was *my* mother staring back at me! *I looked like my mother!* Not that that was terrible, my mother was a very attractive woman, however, she *was* forty years older than me. I tried not to panic. At least it wasn't my *grandmother* staring back at me! In my research, I discovered that a woman's skin *is indeed* affected in perimenopause and there are many skin changes that can occur. Lowered estrogen levels influence the amount of collagen present in the skin and as a result the skin becomes less elastic and thinner. The aging progression also contributes to skin alterations as follows: (1) The skin restores old cells at a slower pace with age, hence there is less turnover of surface skin. (2) Skin cells repair themselves less efficiently with age, hence slower wound healing. (3) The oil-producing glands of the skin are less active with age, hence drier skin. And, (4) the protective layer of subcutaneous fat decreases with age, hence the skin becomes thinner and more delicate, offering less resilience.[77] A woman's diet, medication regime/history, medical history, genetics, the amount of lifetime sun exposure, living environment history, work environment history, stress level, stress history, and smoking history are other important factors that can affect her skin tone.

In the dead of night, one really late night, as I was watching television (I couldn't get back to sleep), I realized that almost every other commercial on T.V. had to do with skin creams, skin lotions, and/or tools and techniques to help retain and restore a youthful appearance. Tight, taut skin was definitely in! No matter *what* station I turned on, I was bombarded with these advertisements, infomercials, and testimonials about skin care products that rejuvenated and lifted the skin. A wrinkle, no matter how small, was perceived as a horrible phenomenon that had to be dealt with at any cost, and hopefully, erased by whatever means necessary. The message that I took away from the many ads and infomercials I viewed that night was simple; In this culture you didn't want to show even the *slightest* sign of aging. With so much emphasis on youth and maintaining a youthful appearance in our society, it is easy to conclude that cultural biases are *indeed* largely to blame for putting pressure on and lowering self esteem in the aging, perimenopausal woman. There are not only societal demands for preserving youth and physical fitness, but also for maintaining a youthful attitude and a young-at-heart outlook on life.[78] How can the aging perimenopausal woman *ever* compete in this youth-oriented society? And, why should she even have to? What is so dreadful about looking and acting one's age???

Another skin change that may crop up in perimenopause is an itchy, crawly sensation under the skin. Formication (no, not *fornication* which means something else totally different) is the bizarre feeling that ants are crawling on the skin. This has actually been estimated to occur in approximately 20% of perimenopausal women. An electric shock sensation under the skin or in the head and a tingling sensation in the extremities are other skin sensations that have also been reported by some perimenopausal women.

Appearing as fifteen on the list of losses, there may be **a loss of or a change in hair color, quantity, texture, and/or luster**. Around the time of middle age, many of us, both men and women, will probably start to observe our head and body hair **turn another color**—a shade of gray or white. It is believed that genetics primarily determine when this particular event happens.[79] The pigment (color) cells at the base of the hair follicle stop producing melanin, i.e. hair minus melanin = gray/white hair. The melanin that is responsible for hair color is actually produced for *each* individual strand of hair which is the reason why hair appears to turn gray or white strand-by-individual-strand. Gray hair still has some pigment present, but white tresses have *no* pigment present. Gray or white hair seems to be a **different texture** too. It is much coarser than the manes of younger years, and sometimes it seems to have a mind of its own! Interestingly, gray hair appears earlier in Whites and later in Asians.

Furthermore, some **hair loss** may be observed during this phase of life. There are several theories for this as follows: (1) Hair loss is likely hormonally related in women due to declines in estrogen levels. (2) New hair growth slows down at this point in life resulting in thinner hair.[80] (3) Some pattern hair loss is thought to be connected to the immune system. Male hormones, especially DHT, may cause an autoimmune response that starts an attack on the hair follicle. (4) Genetics may be a contributing factor (or causative agent) in some hair loss. (5) Certain medical conditions may cause hair loss, e.g. thyroid disease, iron-deficient anemia, lupus, and other infections.[81] (6) Certain medications may cause hair loss, e.g. heparin, high dose aspirin therapy, some cancer medications/treatments, anti-thyroid medications, etc.[82] Finally, (7) stress may be responsible for hair loss in certain instances, but the hair usually grows back within a year of eliminating the stressor(s).[83]

The perimenopausal woman may also notice a change in her hair's **luster**. I noticed that my hair started looking very lackluster. It was not the same shiny, bouncy mane I'd known in pervious years. Apparently, drab looking hair in mid-life occurs because of (1) the hormonal changes in perimenopause, and (2) the hair shafts begin to thin and dry.[84]

Can you believe this list of losses in perimenopause is still unfolding? Sixteenth, there may be a **loss of self image, therefore a negative self image may develop and/or there may be a loss of body image, therefore a negative body image may develop**. Self image and body image can be positive or negative. **Self image** is the mental perception that an individual has of herself or himself (how one sees oneself).[85] It includes the individual's assessment of her own character, the individual's perception of how she believes others perceive her, personality, accomplishments in academics and athletics,[86] skills, knowledge, abilities, body image, relationships,[87] background,[88] goals,[89] accumulated scripts,[90] values, and personal worth.[91] Self image is also influenced by internal monologue (or self talk). Unfortunately, research has shown that almost 87% of self talk about ourselves is negative!!![92] And finally, self image may also vary greatly from the way others perceive the individual.

Given that body image is so closely related to self image, the physical changes occurring during perimenopause and the affects of the aging process can result in a woman feeling unsure of herself, uncomfortable, and/or unhappy with her new physical appearance. And, since perimenopause *does* parallel mid-life, many women will implement a self-inventory, as stated in the ninth loss. This is a time of introspection and reflection on the past. If the perimenopausal woman is not at ease with the choices, outcomes, achievements, accomplishments, and/or the woman she has become, then she may also develop a negative self-image.

**Body image**, one element of self-image, is how an individual feels about the way she/he looks.[93] In other words, body image is the mental perception that an individual has of her outer appearance. It includes body size, body shape, and general appearance.[94] Body image actually develops early on via social interaction with others, it is feedback driven, and it continually changes throughout the lifespan.[95] There are many factors responsible in determining one's body image. Prevailing social standards, socialization, self-esteem, others' reactions, observations, or remarks (this could also include abuse—physical, mental, sexual, discrimination, or harassment), and physical life-altering events, i.e. puberty, pregnancy, and menopause are all factors that determine body image.[96]

With all of the changes that a woman may experience during perimenopause affecting her physical appearance, i.e. muscle mass decreases, body fat increases, weight fluctuations/gains/redistributions, skin changes, breast changes, hair changes, etc. it becomes easy for her to develop insecurity and a lack of confidence in her physical appearance. At this point, a negative body image may develop. Remember that body image is modified throughout the lifespan. And, just as the adolescent girl discovers a new physical appearance, resulting in body image changes, so too the perimenopausal woman discovers a new physical appearance that results in body image changes. Research indicates that women, in general, are much more critical of their appearance than men anyway.[97] And, with so much emphasis on preserving a youthful, wrinkle-free, thin appearance in this society, there is an *enormous* pressure and stress on the perimenopausal woman to look and perform as she did in previous years. Now, I am *not* saying that a perimenopausal woman should let herself go, or that perimenopause is an excuse to let herself go, but I *am* saying that there is an excessive youth-oriented, physical, and sexual emphasis that exists in this culture today that places unrealistic and unnecessary expectations on the aging woman.

The seventeenth loss involves a **loss of breast mass**. I began noticing that my size "A" breasts were shrinking!

*My God, I will be in a girl's training bra by the time this over!* I thought. I was so small to begin with, and here they were disappearing more each day right before my eyes! I wouldn't have minded half as much if my hips were equally as small, but they weren't. This was particularly shocking to me as I *never* thought my chest would shrink as I aged. I discovered that with decreased circulating estrogen levels in perimenopause, the breasts do become fattier and less dense (note: dense is more stromal and epithelial tissue, rather than fat). And, a loss of elasticity may result in the breasts drooping and they may also become flatter.[98] Some women perceive this particular loss as a deficit to their womanhood and femininity. I certainly wasn't real thrilled about losing the little bit that I had. The body that I had learned to live with for the past thirty $^+$ years since adolescence was transforming into something much different than what I had become accustomed to. It was really scary. What would the end result be?

A woman may have had *no* problem whatsoever maintaining a stable weight throughout her life only to find that now she *cannot* keep the extra pounds off. A **loss of weight control** may alter a woman's body during perimenopause in the eighteenth loss. Is the weight gain from the aging process itself? Increased food intake? Less physical activity? Or, hormonal fluctuations? Evidently, there are actual **physical causes** to blame for increased weight gain at this time of life. The physical nature of some weight gain in perimenopause has to do with brain chemical fluctuations. Neurotransmitters, such as serotonin, can fluctuate causing food cravings. For instance, cravings for carbs like potatoes, white bread, or pasta may increase. In fact, the average woman will gain 10–12 pounds during the menopause phase.[99] And, compared to other women of other ages, post menopausal women *do* have more body fat than younger women. However, there are other reasons for weight gain during perimenopause and beyond. With declining ovarian estrogen production in perimenopause, the body's fat cells start producing supplemental estrogen. And…just guess where many of these fat cells are located? In the abdominal area. Pooch! It is also very interesting that the three principal hormonal transitions in a woman's lifespan (menarche, childbirth, and menopause) are correlated with changes in body fat distribution.[100]

Even though there are hormonal influences and other physiological changes responsible for weight gain, perimenopause, and finally menopause, occur at a time when the **aging process** itself is also contributing to a slower metabolic rate and a decrease in overall muscle mass. It has been suggested that caloric needs in mid-life can drop by as much as 400–500 calories per day! As we age, we also become **less active**. And, exercise may become problematic too, especially if there are physical limitations. For me, on the days when I was experiencing joint aches, I certainly wasn't in a rush to exercise. It becomes difficult to tease out one cause from the other (perimenopause vs. aging) to blame for weight gain in this phase of life. Weight gain may very well be a result of both of these life events happening simultaneously.

In the nineteenth loss, there may be a temporary **loss of overall physical well being and/or a decreased quality of life** with all of the aches and pains that can accompany perimenopause. The many physical and psychological signs a woman may experience during perimenopause can easily become a negative influence on her activities of daily living (ADL's)☺. She may experience any or all of the losses mentioned in this chapter affecting her physical and psychological health and/or she may experience generalized fatigue. For myself, in addition to the joint pain that I was experiencing, I was beginning to experience *horrific* migraine headaches on a regular basis. I would call these headaches "hormone headaches" because no matter *what* I did to treat them, they just would not go away. And…I *knew* they were hormonally related because of the time of onset and duration. Many nights I would go to bed with a pounding sensation in my head, usually located over one of my eyes, only to wake up with it again the next morning, only worse! The affected eye would throb and even water, the headaches were so bad. Watching television or even having any lights on around me would make me nauseous in classic migraine style. I *never* had headaches of this magnitude before, and any headache I did have, would usually disappear within a few hours of taking some Tylenol or aspirin. These "hormone" headaches were definitely debilitating and would hold me down for hours, even days. My research revealed that there *is* evidence suggesting a significant relationship between migraine headaches and **estrogen** (**dominance**\*). A headache can happen as the CNS responds to hormonal fluctuations (not their presence, but fluctuations). Also, with the hormonal variations in perimenopause, existing headaches can actually intensify or new headaches or headache patterns can emerge. It was interesting to find out that the *highest* incidence of migraines actually occurs in women approximately forty years of age.[101] Fortunately, after menopause, the incidence of migraines declines.[102] This fact would certainly seem to indicate that hormonal involvement is undoubtedly linked to migraine headaches

\***Estrogen Dominance** is a state where greater levels of estrogen are present compared to circulating progesterone levels. This event can occur in perimenopause due to a progesterone production reduction (in the ovaries). Other reasons for estrogen dominance include HT, stress, obesity, high levels of environmental xenoestrogens☺, and estrogens consumed from hormone fed cattle and poultry, to name a few, according to Dr. Michael Lam, a specialist in nutritional and anti-aging medicine.

There seems to be some differences in occurrence of perimenopausal signs within our culture too. Black women, for example, have reported a higher incidence of estrogen-related signs including hot flashes, night sweats, and a change or loss of bladder control. But, this particular ethnic group is also likely to experience *fewer* somatic signs such as headaches, sleep disturbances, palpitations, and aching or stiff joints.[103, 104] There are ethnic differences in the occurrence of osteoporosis too, according to The National Osteoporosis Foundation as illustrated in the following chart (listed in order of incidence):

| Ethnicity | Percent Estimated to have Osteoporosis | Percent Estimated to have Low Bone Mass |
|---|---|---|
| White and Asian women Non-Hispanic Aged 50 and up | 20% | 52% |
| Hispanic women Aged 50 and up | 10% | 49% |
| Black women Non-Hispanic Aged 50 and up | 5% | 35% |

I was also experiencing some extreme dizziness at times which definitely affected my daily living. Luckily, I was busy at home working on this book, so if I did feel woozy I could lie down on the couch until the feeling passed. There didn't seem to be any pattern to the vertigo-like wooziness and I initially thought my diet was to blame. But, after modifying my diet, and changing the times of day I ate, there was no impact whatsoever on the dizziness that I was experiencing. Other women shared with me that they too experienced dizziness at times during the perimenopause process and some of them continued experiencing dizziness for ten to fifteen years after menopause.

Number twenty on the list of losses may include a **loss of confidence in decision-making ability**. I had always been a focused person with a great deal of self assurance in my decisions for most of my life. I quickly and effortlessly made decisions in all aspects of my life. However, more recently, I found myself hesitant and *extremely* over-cautious in every single choice that I made. Part of the problem was, in my mind anyway, the fact that now that I was here in middle age, there was no time left to mess up any more. If I *did* make a poor decision, especially one that cost me money, I didn't feel as if I had a whole lot of time left to recoup the loss. Whereas, if I made sorry choices in my twenties and thirties (which we all do), there was much more time remaining to cover the losses. Now any extra finances needed to be directed toward my future, particularly retirement, and not toward recovering from some seriously impulsive, clumsy choices.

So…I ended up analyzing *everything* to death before I could formulate any sort of solid decision, which resulted in time-consuming, drawn out, yet very carefully selected choices that protected my future. Paradoxically, in one respect, I *had* lost self confidence in my decision-making ability because of the time element involved, and yet, I was actually becoming very skilled in the art of decision-making, carefully weighing the pros and cons of each and every choice. At this point though, it became difficult for me to make quick, immediate decisions, which could be a serious deficit when I integrated back into the workforce, where hasty decisions were required on a day-to-day basis.

Remember that every woman experiences perimenopause uniquely. This particular alteration in my behavior may *only* apply to a few women, as I had actually heard other women commenting that with age they felt more confident than ever before with their decision-making ability. With me though, I ended up questioning everything and then checking it twice. However, I must say that I *was* very comfortable with my "final decision".

The twenty-first and final loss in perimenopause consists of **miscellaneous losses**. A woman has reached a time in her life where she not only has to face the losses that occur during her own personal perimenopause, but she must confront other major life events and/or losses that may also occur now. (Some of these are discussed in the next chapter in more detail.) For instance, she may have aging, sick parents who pass on. She may lose a child or children to college, marriage, or some other living arrangement. She may lose a significant other/spouse to a split, separation, divorce, or even death. Many families acquire pets while their children are young and as the child grows, the pet ages too. Thus, she may encounter an aging/sick pet or even lose a cherished family pet at this time. Or, she may lose a certain lifestyle with a relocation or the sale of an existing home that suddenly becomes too large when a child or children leave home. Finally, the loss of family members and/or friends due to a split/divorce/illness/death can result in a very important loss, namely the loss of a woman's support system. And, this loss comes at a time when a woman truly needs a strong support network.

At the other end of the continuum, if a woman has delayed starting a family until she is in her forties, or she finds herself caring for an elderly or ill parent, in-law, or other family member, then she may find herself upscaling to accommodate others, i.e. she may need more space in the house, a larger automobile, etc.

In retrospection, isn't it *amazing* how many losses a woman can encounter during perimenopause? And, I am sure there are other losses not even covered here. In my research, I came across many professionals rejecting the concept of loss altogether during the menopause transition. It is my individual female experience however, that there *are* losses/issues/concerns (whatever you want to call them). I have experienced these losses first-hand. And, so what? Do we travel on this journey of life never experiencing loss? Of course not, as explained earlier. Therefore, it is important to recognize these losses and to process the grief to be able to move on. Unfortunately, many women seem to stumble through the perimenopausal process experiencing these losses and experiencing the emotion not really knowing what is happening to them. And, most of us probably don't even consider the psychological impact that these losses can have, yet these losses are *so* instrumental in shaping a woman's individuality.

Lastly, in the final stages of the grieving process, acceptance and resolution are ultimately achieved. So…many of the losses that *do* occur during perimenopause will eventually be accepted and resolved. And, there are many gains that can offset the losses and they are discussed in detail in the next chapter.

As a final point, some losses *can* be intervened or delayed, i.e. skin care products/tools/techniques and surgical or non-surgical intervention can improve skin tone/appearance. HT or BHRT can replace diminished estrogen and progesterone levels restoring many of the benefits of these hormones. Supplemental testosterone can help restore and maintain a strong libido. Surgical intervention can enhance or lift the breasts. Hair coloring, highlighting, weaving, or other techniques can restore tresses back to its original color, thickness, and/or texture. Psychotherapy, support groups, diet, or exercise can assist with a negative body or self image, and so on. The point is women *do* have options in managing the individual losses and changes that can occur during the perimenopause process (note: this will be discussed further in the next chapter, specifically in the sixth gain).

# 4

# *Let Me Count the Gains*

Is it any wonder that there is grieving and/or mourning during perimenopause in view of all of the aforementioned losses that can occur? When I actually saw all of the losses spelled out, it left me wondering. *There has to be some advantage here.* I considered. *It can't be all bad.*

And, as I continued on my quest for information and enlightenment on the topic of perimenopause, I realized that accompanying these perimenopausal losses *were* many gains that did seem to outweigh any discomforts, inconveniences, and changes that could happen during perimenopause. I discovered that there is indeed an *enormous* personal growth potential here through specific gains that by far overshadows any negative perimenopausal signs. Ultimately, beyond the menopause metamorphosis, there emerges a more confident, self-assured woman who is better equipped in her decision-making ability, more prioritized about her life, more relaxed, more laid back, and she will probably be happier and more content with herself than she has ever been before. And, her physical appearance and physical fitness can actually be improved as well.

Now I am not talking about "weight gains" here. I am talking about the psychological and spiritual development, wisdom, knowledge, and maturation that takes place, not *only* as a result of perimenopause, but also as a result of a life experience that is at the approximate half-way point (considering the current American female lifespan of 79.8 years that increases every decade).[105] And, I am talking about gains like the physical and psychological freedom from a monthly cycle. And, the physical and psychological freedom from birth control needs and concerns, etc. **Perimenopause is merely a vehicle that drives a woman down the road of personal development**. If a woman does not purposely decelerate her vehicle through denial, stubbornness, or uncooperativeness with the entire perimenopause process, then she can accelerate through this middle stretch of life with *great* momentum. Some women completely deny and/or totally disregard the fact that mid-life and with it perimenopause have approached, and they in turn ignore how important these mid-life events are for their future success, happiness, and development.

Why should a woman look forward to perimenopause? And, why should our society review its current pessimistic perception of menopause and assume a more positive position, focusing on the gains and not the losses? There really is a simple answer to both of these questions. Plainly speaking, it is **because there are *so* many *positive* changes and gains to look forward to during perimenopause, at menopause, and especially in post menopause**. Below, the gains a woman may experience during this time of life are discussed. Once again, there is no preference to the order in which they are discussed and one gain is not necessarily more important than another gain. Most women will experience some of the benefits of perimenopause listed below, but because the perimenopause experience is so individualized, each woman will discover her own unique mix of gains.

First on the list of gains, it is likely that a woman will **gain an understanding or gain specific knowledge of her future goals, aspirations, and objectives through reflection on her past**. This is a time when the past becomes *extremely* valuable in the lessons it has offered. With the mid-life introspection that usually accompanies perimenopause, a woman will be sorting through past performance and outcomes, the quality of past and present personal relationships, her child's/ children's success, her education, her career, her hobbies, her home, her finances, her assets, and anything else that involves her life in an attempt to better map out future goals and aspirations. This mid-life introspection emerges in men as well around the same time as it does in women. In some cases, this event may initially surface as sporadic and fleeting thoughts, reflections, or feelings and the woman may be totally unaware of what is happening. But, as time goes on, and these reflective thoughts and feelings become more frequent and intense (sometimes even intrusive), a woman will eventually realize that a sort of mid-life assessment is occurring. I noticed that many profound, philosophical thoughts would pop into my mind when I was driving in my car. It could be that when I was driving, although I was focused on the road, the traffic signs, the traffic lights, the cars in front of me, the cars behind me, etc., I was alone and I had time to think.

Once this mid-life assessment has begun, a woman is actually better prepared to make decisions concerning her future. For example, she may not want to continue on the same career path that she has been on when she realizes that she has been performing in the same job position for years and has not attained the status or the wages she really wanted. Or, she may decide to move on from an unhealthy relationship that she has maintained for way too long. Or, she may decide to relocate, etc. And so, the mid-life introspection assists mid-lifers in planning for the future and hopefully assists them in modifying the road to personal success (whatever that may be).

Second, as a result of the above-mentioned mid-life evaluation that takes place, a woman **will gain awareness that her life has reached the approximate half-way mark**. This is an *extremely* important growth tool in that the **time element** remaining in her lifespan is now recognized. The time that we actually have on this earth was not a consideration in our teens, in our twenties, or even in our thirties. In those younger years, we considered the rest of lives to be "forever". And, some of the choices we made back then certainly reflected that relaxed attitude! However, now that mid-life has arrived, there is not as much time left to achieve our goals and to recoup any emotional or financial losses we may have suffered. Time *suddenly* becomes a very valuable commodity. And, many of us realize that the time we *do* have left should be valued and cherished.

So…for example, even though a perimenopausal woman may experience a loss of confidence in her decision-making ability (loss #20), **she *will* benefit from this "time element" awareness that can positively affect her decision-making skills**. "Time element awareness" teaches us that we cannot waste precious time and/or resources making impulsive and ultimately poor decisions at this stage in the lifespan. The recognition that there is a finite amount of time remaining on our clocks helps us in planning our futures, i.e. retirement is not far away for a woman in her late forties or early fifties If a financial retirement plan has not been established at this point, there are only so many working years left to make the plan rock solid enough to retire on comfortably. And, in this unstable economy in which we presently live, it is even *more* difficult to plan for the future. I know several people who drained their entire retirement account to support themselves during periods of unemployment or illness. Or, they lived off the money that they were able to obtain from equity loans/lines of credit on their homes, leaving them with little or no equity in their homes for the future. This becomes a serious problem when retirement is only a few years away.

This **time element awareness or mortality awareness** that occurs during perimenopause may occur not only as a result of time component consideration, but it may also occur from the woman's experience with negative perimenopausal signs that can cause her to become more aware of her own physical limits and temporal finiteness. It is also possible that she may reach this new awareness simply by observing how aging or ill family members, friends, or even pets deal with their own mortality.

Third on the list of gains, a woman will most likely **experience a priority assessment and/or a priority shift**. For the majority of us (men included), a priority assessment and/or a priority shift will occur during mid-life, a time that parallels a woman's perimenopause. With the realization that the number of days on this earth are numbered, a middle-aged woman will begin to prioritize and reorganize her life, and/or her priorities will undergo a transformation—sometimes a drastic transformation. Things that she once thought were red hot important, are clearly not that important now. Priority assessment and/or priority shifting can occur at other times during the lifespan too. For example, when we reach a certain age that is significant for us (which is different for each individual—for me it was thirty), or we reach a certain place in life, i.e. graduation, new/different career, new/different job, new/different living arrangement, a new/special relationship, marriage, divorce, illness, death, birth, etc., we realize that: (1) we must grow up, (2) we must become independent, (3) we must make changes, (4) we must become better, etc. And, these significant life events force us to reassess things as they are. When a child is born for instance, and we look into the tiny little being's pure, bright eyes, we quickly realize that the things we once considered to be sizzling with importance, suddenly take a back seat to the child and to his/her happiness/comfort. As painful as this mid-life priority assessment and/or priority shifting can be, it is extremely beneficial in helping us to successfully plan for our futures. It makes us stop in our tracks and think.

One of these mid-life priority shifts that I experienced involved my car. I purchased a brand new BMW for myself back in 1992. What an *awesome* feeling it was driving that spanking new BMW off the car lot! I opened the sunroof to feel the warm Florida sun on my skin and let the breeze play with my hair as I drove my new BMW home that day. It was *definitely* "the ultimate driving machine"! It was by far the best performing and the most comfortable car I had ever owned. I really loved that car until four years later when some kid plowed into me with his wreck of a car, totaling my beautiful BMW. For many years, I dreamed of being able to purchase another new BMW. But, one thing or another always sidetracked me financially. I returned to college. My son needed new bedroom furniture. I was downsized. Our fridge broke. We needed a new washing machine, etc. It *never* ended! And, I *never* did get another new BMW. However, upon entering mid-life and experiencing this priority shift, I finally realized that a new BMW was not in the cards anymore and the twelve year old car that I was currently driving would have to suffice. I was approaching retirement age too quickly and any extra money I did have needed to be directed toward my daily survival and then retirement, not a new car. My priorities had totally shifted.

In the fourth gain, a woman who has approached perimenopause **has successfully gained entrance into a *huge* milestone in her lifespan**. There are *many* milestones in the human experience that could be considered momentous and that can be critical turning points. In my case, I am not sure why, or exactly what significance a particular age has, but when I turned thirty, it seemed like a real turning point in my life and I felt very proud to have made it that far. Another life experience that I considered momentous was when my only son reached his first birthday. I was *so* elated that he had made it and that he was now walking, talking, and running! As a mother, I was filled with pride that day.

*I must have done everything right to get him here!* I happily contemplated, watching him stuff *way* too much chocolate birthday cake into his tiny mouth. His very first birthday was one milestone, as a mother, I will never forget.

Any woman should be *filled* with a sense of satisfaction and appreciation that she has even arrived at this particular life event called perimenopause. Let's face it—fifty years on this earth in this place called "life" is definitely worth celebrating! It marks the beginning of the end of the reproductive years, the approximate mid point in the lifespan, and the beginning of a totally new experience for a woman that will continue on for another thirty or so years. And so, there are demarcations in one's lifespan that signify an important, and sometimes life altering event has arrived. Perimenopause is one these events.

With the signs, discomforts, distresses, weight gains and shifts, and other changes that can accompany perimenopause, a woman will probably become acutely aware of her physical body at this time. So…fifth, a woman will **gain the advantage of being totally tuned into her physical being**. Typically in our society, we carry on with our busy daily routines, maybe not making the best food choices, not exercising as we should, not following a skin care regimen, etc. until one day our bodies scream for "Help"! This cry for "Help" may very well be heard during perimenopause when there are other physiological changes occurring that *require* us to respond, i.e. loss/declines in sex hormones (loss #3 and #7), etc. that surface as perimenopausal signs. When we start noticing differences in our bodies, we become *very* aware, sometimes *painfully* aware of what it is trying to tell us. We don't have a choice at this point but *to* listen! Even though hormonal fluctuations and declines are partially responsible for perimenopausal signs, our physical health is also essentially a product of what we do to it on a daily basis and what we have done to it up to this point.

The time of perimenopause can, in fact, be a time when a woman becomes the *most* health conscious and consequently the healthiest. Some women will actually start a regimented physical health routine by increasing the amount of exercise and/or redefining eating habits during these perimenopausal years in an effort to maintain or regain physical fitness. A perimenopausal woman may realize, with the addition of a few extra pounds, that her metabolism is starting to slow down. Or, she may notice weight redistribution in specific areas. Or, she may realize that her stamina is starting to wane, for instance, as she becomes short-winded and fatigued climbing a set of stairs that she had no problem climbing before. Perimenopause is an ideal time for a woman to evaluate her physical condition and make the necessary modifications to keep her feeling vibrant and energetic. Exercise is *key* to staying in shape, keeping the weight down, and maintaining strong muscles and healthy bones. Exercise also increases the body's metabolic rate, therefore the body burns more calories. And, strength training can actually improve muscle mass and affect bones positively. I don't think *anyone* could despise exercise more than me! But…I realized that exercise was a key component to good health and weight management. I found that by walking as much as I could and then doing weight training and stretching on the days that I couldn't walk was actually invigorating. I had more energy and I slept better.

Furthermore, if a woman has been burning the candle at both ends, like so many women today (career women, supermoms, caretakers), she might have to slow down and start taking care of herself, especially if her body is telling her to do so. Currently in our society, many women are *extremely* driven, sometimes not by choice, and they, in turn, may end up working long hours by holding several jobs. In fact, today many women hold more than one job outside the home. They may have a career outside the home and a family in the home to care for. They may have caretaker duties caring for an elderly or ill parent, another family member, or a pet. They may be attending college full-time, or attending college and working too. A woman must wear many different hats nowadays and it may become difficult for her to slow down once the pace is set. The point here is for the perimenopausal woman to pay attention to and listen to what the physical self is communicating and adjust accordingly.

In the sixth gain, a woman will **gain the knowledge that she does have control managing her perimenopause via a variety of options**. In an effort to take charge of the perimenopausal signs that can crop up, a woman will probably become cognizant of the fact (through education, communication with others, media, etc.) that she does have a variety of options available to her in managing her perimenopausal signs. In my opinion, the options available to her today could be improved, but at least she has many more choices than in the past. Even though she may feel that she has *totally* lost control of herself with all of the changes that may be affecting her, there is still some power she can maintain in the form of personal perimenopause management choices. Remember that every woman's perimenopausal experience is unique, so each woman will have a different set of concerns or needs in handling her own individual perimenopause. Some of the tools available to women today that can assist in managing, influencing, controlling, and coping with perimenopause are mentioned below. Other options are available, but I have tried to capture the main ones here.

1. **Education**: By exposing herself to as much information as possible, the perimenopausal woman will be correctly and accurately informed about the entire perimenopause process. She will be more comfortable with and accepting of what to expect and how to manage her perimenopause. There are numerous ways of getting information on the topic. These include books, magazines, television, radio, internet, other individuals, support groups, health care providers, etc. And, there are resources listed at the end of this book (*Additional Perimenopause Resources*). You are *already* reading this book, so you are off to a great start!

2. **Attitude**: A positive attitude can assist a woman's passage through perimenopause by allowing her to focus on the positive aspects of perimenopause, i.e. personal growth, development, freedom from monthly inconveniences and birth control concerns, etc. and not dwell on the negative aspects of perimenopause such as joint aches, hot flashes, moodiness, etc. An optimistic outlook can also help a woman better manage and cope with any negative signs that she may be experiencing with more confidence. And, a positive attitude can help her to willingly receive and accept the entire perimenopause experience instead of dreading it.

3. **Communication**: I cannot stress this more—communication with others is *key* to an easy and successful journey through perimenopause. Others' personal experiences and individual stories about perimenopause can offer the perimenopausal woman invaluable insight into the perimenopause progression. However, even though I strongly advocate seeking information from other women, this should *not* be the only resource the perimenopausal woman consults. Since every woman's experience with perimenopause is different, each woman will only be able to offer limited pieces of information. An assortment of other sources that are reliable and complete in content should also be explored so that a *total* picture of the perimenopause transformation is captured. You will find some of the resources that I found very helpful listed at the end of the book (*Additional Perimenopause Resources*).

4. **Hormone Therapy (HT)**: HT supplies a woman with the female sex hormones that gradually diminish with age.[106] Until recently, almost 40% of post

menopausal women in this country used HT.[107] However, that number is changing with the recent HT controversy. Traditional HT is synthetically produced.
When estrogen is the only hormone given, it is referred to as Estrogen Replacement Therapy (ERT), when progestin is combined with estrogen, then it is
referred to as Hormone Therapy (HT), previously referred to as Hormone
Replacement Therapy (HRT).[108] Why take HT? HT can improve the quality of
life for some women by relieving particular negative signs of perimenopause, e.g.
hot flashes, sleep difficulties, vaginal dryness, etc. and HT can help prevent
osteoporosis and other illnesses.[109] Women should be aware though that HT has
recently become very controversial in that the largest clinical studies in the U.S.,
The National Institutes of Health's (NIH)☺Women's Health Initiative (WHI),
halted a major clinical trial early due to the increased risk of invasive breast cancer
in women from HT.[110] There was also an increased risk of heart disease, stroke,
and blood clots. And, the study also indicated that ERT appeared to increase the
risk of stroke.[111] Even though HT is still available, a woman must *strongly* consider the benefits vs. the risks before taking any hormone therapy.

5. **Bioidentical Hormone Replacement Therapy (BHRT)**☺: BHRT supplies
a woman with the female sex hormones that are declining with age. BHRT can be
extracted from plants, (soy, yams), animals (pigs, horses), or they can be synthetically produced[112] and through chemical processes they are converted to human
hormones.[113] Bioidentical hormones have the exact molecular structure as those
made in the human body and they have the same physiologic responses as endoge-
nous hormones.[114] The greatest benefit of BHRT is that they are more natural than
HT and they are customized to *each* individual's needs by a compounding pharmacist who prepares the product from a physician's prescription. However, a woman
needs to be cautioned before taking BHRT. Even though BHRT is considered by
some to be a safer therapy for perimenopausal, menopausal, and post menopausal
women, no real safety trials have yet been conducted.[115]

6. **Natural Progesterone**: Natural Progesterone supplies a woman with the
hormone progesterone that gradually tapers off as a woman ages. Remember that
progesterone levels decrease in menopause. As mentioned earlier, progesterone
levels diminish to almost *zero* in menopause.[116] Natural Progesterone can also
help balance an estrogen dominant state, it can increase bone density, and it can
improve cardiovascular health.[117] Natural progesterone is *not* the same compound as progestin, progestogen, or other synthetic compounds found in birth
control pills and HT, but it is produced from the wild yam and soybean and it is

believed by some to be the better treatment for negative perimenopausal signs.[118] Again, women must be cautioned that no human clinical trials have really been conducted. Project AWARE has a great synopsis of the hormone progesterone. See the end of this book *Additional Perimenopause Resources* for their web site.

7. **Herbs**: Herbs may be utilized during perimenopause to relieve negative perimenopausal signs, boost energy levels, and to assist in overall well health. Herbs act on the pituitary gland, the ovaries, and estrogen-dependent cells to reduce negative perimenopausal signs such as hot flashes, mood swings, etc.[119] Some women may feel more confident using herb therapy as opposed to HT or BHRT as: (1) Herbs have successfully been used for centuries by different peoples. (2) Herbs offer a natural alternative to synthetically produced treatment or chemical treatment. And, (3) herbs do not have certain side effects that traditional pharmacological treatments may have.[120] Women should be aware though that some herbs may interfere with or even intensify certain medications' actions and a professional should be consulted before starting herbal therapy.[121]

8. **Nutrition**: Perimenopause, menopause, and post menopause create some unique dietary requirements in women in that (1) the metabolic rate is slowing down, (2) muscle mass is decreasing, (3) bone mass begins to decline, (4) energy and stamina levels decline, (5) the skin is drier, (6) hair becomes lackluster, etc. These changes produce specific nutritional needs that start during perimenopause. Foods high in calcium or calcium supplements should be started now. Hydration should not be overlooked. And, some women may feel better during perimenopause if they eat smaller amounts of food more frequently, as a drop in blood glucose levels may actually increase some negative perimenopausal signs.[122]

9. **Exercise**: Exercise offers many positive benefits to a woman during perimenopause. It can decrease negative perimenopausal signs such as anxiety and sleep disturbances, and it has been found that women who exercise appear to have fewer hot flashes than women who don't exercise.[123] In fact, being sedentary may actually *increase* the incidence of hot flashes during perimenopause,[124] being sedentary may lead to back pain, and being sedentary may cause stiffness.[125] Exercise can decrease or delay signs of aging,[126] it can promote cardiovascular fitness (by affecting blood pressure, blood fats, cholesterol, and blood glucose),[127] and weight bearing exercises can strengthen bones, i.e. exercise stimulates bones to retain the minerals that keep them dense.[128] Exercise has a positive effect on moods too, i.e. endorphins are released in the brain.[129] Finally, the Kegel exercise

can strengthen the pelvic floor muscles which affect the bladder, urethra, uterus, vagina, and rectum.[130]

10. **Yoga:** Yoga techniques can help alleviate negative perimenopausal signs a woman may be experiencing and help in her overall well health and attitude through exercise, stretching, and meditation. Meditation can help ease irritability, mood swings, and depression, and other exercises can improve a woman's circulation, assist in balancing metabolism, and prevent memory loss.[131]

11. **Acupuncture:** Acupuncture is the ancient Chinese treatment that can help reduce negative perimenopausal signs such as hot flashes, insomnia, and nervousness by rebalancing the hormonal system.[132] Acupuncture stimulates (with fine gauge needles—the width of two human hairs)[133] certain pressure points (points that are located near or on the surface of the skin) that then alters the body's biochemical and physiological elements decreasing negative perimenopausal signs.[134] The needles are believed to encourage the flow of "Qi" (chee) or natural healing energy.[135] Treatment will probably include several sessions.[136] Studies conducted in the late 90's by Dr. Susan Cohen D.S.N. APRN, Associate Professor of the University of Pittsburgh, revealed that acupuncture did indeed decrease hot flashes by 35% and decreased insomnia by 50%.[137] Women may choose this particular method of reducing negative perimenopausal signs because it has successfully been used since approximately 3A.D. and it is an individualized treatment.[138]

12. **Acupressure:** Acupressure is a form of healing treatment based on ancient Japanese and Chinese medicine[139] that can be used during perimenopause to reduce negative signs such as hot flashes, by encouraging the body's own healing energy. Acupressure is similar to acupuncture in that it treats energy blockages except that acupressure uses applied pressure (usually with the fingers) and not needles to specific points on the body.[140] Acupressure helps stimulate the ovaries, uterus, adrenals, pituitary, thyroid and parathyroid glands which can assist in balancing the hormonal system.[141] According to *Alternative Therapies in Health and Medicine* (July 11, 2001), one study showed that acupressure did significantly reduce the number of hot flashes in menopausal women.[142]

13. **Address the Signs:** There are numerous aches, pains, and discomforts that may develop during perimenopause. Joint aches, headaches (tension, hormone, or migraine), abdominal pain, vaginal discomfort during intercourse, etc. are some of the discomforts a woman might encounter during perimenopause. Once

the perimenopausal woman has ascertained that there is no pathology involved, certain pain reducing/comfort measures can help alleviate or decrease the aches/pains/discomforts of perimenopause. In other words, confront the negative perimenopausal signs as they surface. For example, I found that by using a warm "Bed Buddy" on my aching joints, any joint discomforts I was experiencing would subside, even if only temporarily. It also helped reduce the intensity of some of the headaches I was experiencing. A "Bed Buddy" resembles a large white sock that is filled with an organic rice-size material that provides moist heat (microwaveable) for aches and pains and it is also effective for backaches, neckaches, headaches, or cramps. As a cold pack (refrigerated), the Bed Buddy would help reduce any puffiness under my eyes. On a more positive note, some pains actually *diminish* with age; while joint pain seems to increase with age in both women and men, abdominal pains and tension-type headaches seem to *decrease* with age in women.[143] And, the incidence of migraine headaches decreases *considerably* in post menopause.[144]

14. **Psychotherapy**: Individual counseling can offer *tremendous* assistance to a woman during perimenopause. The overwhelming nature of perimenopause and the occurrence of other significant mid-life events may leave a woman feeling depressed, helpless, and/or despondent. A psychotherapist, psychiatrist, counselor, etc. can help the passage through perimenopause by offering professional advice on such topics as coping strategies, life skills, relationship issues, etc. And, when a therapist is simply a good listener, this in itself may be invaluable to the perimenopausal woman. It seems that *many* people have an analyst nowadays anyway and the negative stigma that once existed in seeking help in the psychological realm no longer exists. Spiritual or religious counseling may also offer suggestions, support, or comfort during this time.

15. **Support Groups**: There are all kinds of support groups available to the perimenopausal woman today that can offer: (1) emotional support, (2) education, and (3) allow a platform to share personal experiences and to vent. These groups can be especially helpful if there is little or no family support and/or no other sounding board available. Also available are online support groups, support groups located in the community, and spiritual or religious support groups.

16. **Surgical/non-surgical cosmetic options to delay or intervene perimenopausal signs/losses**: There are many surgical/non-surgical cosmetic options available today that can help intervene the aging process. Chemical or mechanical

methods can resurface aging skin, and botox, collagen, surgical face lifts, and surgical breast enhancement or lifts are only some of the procedures that can change the appearance of aging.[145]

17. **Hair stylist/Colorist**: A good hair stylist/colorist can do wonders for a woman's appearance. It used to be said that a woman over forty should not have hair longer than her shoulders. But, why should an age, a number, dictate a woman's hair style or hair length? What is the difference how long her hair is, as long as it is flattering and neat? Also, a good hair colorist can help restore hair to its original color, or even apply a new color, which can disguise the appearance of aging. However, a woman should avoid over-styling or over-processing her hair, as these can dry the hair and make hair brittle.[146]

18. **Aesthetician**: An aesthetician can assist in delaying the appearance of age on skin tone and skin texture through different techniques and products.

Appearing seventh on the list of gains is something that really took me by surprise. I discovered a **newfound respect and admiration for my mother**! Even though we rarely discussed perimenopause or anything of that nature (it was *always* awkward for me discussing such matters with my mother since her generation didn't seem to discuss topics like this openly), I felt that we actually became closer and our relationship was strengthened. It seems that through the years as we mature, most of us develop a certain respect for our parents, especially for our mothers, and the reality that they have gone through so much to bring us into this world, to feed us, to provide for us, to comfort us, to instill the appropriate values in us, to teach us, and to basically put up with us! Among women, there is a special admiration toward mothers and/or other female family members (sisters, grandmothers, aunts, godmothers, cousins, etc.) and female friends as the exclusive female experiences in adolescence, childbirth, motherhood, menopause, and the aging process occur.

With all of the changes occurring in the perimenopausal woman, this is an *ideal* time to renew old friendships and/or to establish new friendships. Therefore, in the eighth gain, **a woman may gain new relationships during perimenopause**. In contrast to a loss of friends, who may no longer be contributing to her best interests or to her general well being (loss #9), the perimenopausal woman at this time may find herself making new friends who *do* positively contribute to her overall health and happiness. For example, if a new exercise routine is started, say in a gym, on a walking trail, or even in a yoga class, new contacts and ultimately lasting friendships with people sharing the same interests can be created. Also, this may be a time of change with a significant other/spouse via split, separation, divorce, illness, or death. And, a new intimate or close relationship, a new job, a new career, etc. may be in order in which case the perimenopausal woman will have many new connections in her life and the opportunity to form strong, permanent friendships.

With the mid-life evaluation that is taking place, the perimenopausal woman will be reviewing the quality of existing relationships anyway and she may be eliminating some old friendships that are a hindrance to her overall well health, happiness, or life goals (loss #9). Furthermore, friendships the perimenopausal woman may have had with other mothers and other individuals such as teachers, coaches, etc. linked to her child may be diminishing in an empty nest. Once a child graduates from high school and leaves home, relationships with other people connected to the child will most likely face as frequent contact with them decreases.

Appearing ninth on the list of gains in perimenopause, a woman may **gain extra time, flexibility, and/or money**. A woman may find that she now has plenty of extra time, more flexibility to do the things she wants, and/or more money for herself once her child leaves home. Or, she may find more time/flexibility/money after downsizing a larger lifestyle. Or finally, she may find more time and flexibility for herself upon retirement, or from other life circumstances that may also be occurring during this time of life.

So...even though a woman may experience a fading libido during perimenopause (loss #13), she may gain time/conveniences/flexibility/money that actually allow for a better sex life. With many children approaching the age of independence, can you imagine the extra time available, flexibility in location, extra money, and endless possibilities of being able to have sex anywhere, any time? Or, not having to worry about an unwanted pregnancy after menopause? Or, what about a romantic getaway to some exotic location? Lastly, even if the perimenopausal woman is not in the mood, her significant other sure has plenty of flexibility and opportunity now to try to get her in the mood!

Tenth, a perimenopausal woman will **gain mental space and peace of mind in relation to family planning**. With the close of her childbearing years, thoughts of family planning will no longer be on a woman's mind, thus freeing up mental space for other thoughts and allowing a certain peace of mind. How much time do women *really* spend thinking about future offspring? I can remember thinking about how many children I would have (or not have) from the time I was a small girl of five or so playing with dolls. I thought, dreamed, and then talked about having a family countless times with my young girlfriends as they also shared their hopes and dreams with me. And, I revealed my family goals with my adolescent girlfriends as they did with me. I shared my hopes with my parents. I discussed it with men I was seriously involved with. There were *many* thoughts that occupied my mind with how many children to have (or not have), what their names to be, what they would look like, what color hair they would have, what their gender would be, what they would wear, etc.

Additionally, there may be *tremendous* pressure or expectations on a woman from a significant other/spouse, a family member(s), and/or society itself to bear a certain type of child or children. In many cultures and religions, the male child is the preferred gender. A woman is *expected* to bear a male child or children to carry on the family name, to carry on the family business, to carry on family values, etc. Or, a woman may be expected to bear a certain *number* of children. Or, she may be expected to bear a child or children with certain features. This adds an *incredible* amount of pressure on a fertile woman to deliver the goods. With the close of her childbearing years however, these pressures and expectations can at last be alleviated from her thoughts.

As a final thought to gaining peace of mind in relation to family planning—the countless thoughts about that "biological clock" can finally come to an end with the onset of menopause. The clock has stopped ticking!

Eleventh on the list of gains, a woman will **gain the physical freedom from a monthly cycle**. For thirty-five⁺ years a woman has to deal with a monthly cycle and all of the requirements and aggravations that accompany it. I can't *ever* recall another women actually anticipating the monthly cycle unless she was worried about pregnancy. And, what about all the work time, school days, and plans that were changed or lost because she didn't feel well? Accidents, cramps, swelling, headaches, backaches, moodiness, cravings, weight fluctuations/gains, fatigue, pain medications, treatments, and changed or ruined plans are just some of the hassles a woman can *finally* say goodbye to after menopause. Who wouldn't look forward to that?

Twelfth on the list of gains is all of the **psychological liberation, mental space, and peace of mind that is gained by not tending to, thinking about, or worrying about monthly needs, concerns, nuisances, aches, pains, and expenses**. How wonderful! How many times have we women thought about when it would occur, where would we be when it did occur, what time of day would it occur, would we be prepared when it did occur? Someone once told me there should be a bell that rings inside a woman's head when the monthly cycle is about to begin. Unfortunately, we don't have the luxury of having an internal bell or alarm system that goes off in our heads notifying us of the monthly occurrence. So…we guesstimate the best we can. And, there are *many* thoughts spent planning for this monthly event. I remember one job that I had working in a cubicle environment with *all* men surrounding me. Shortly after starting the job, I wondered how I was going to make it to the ladies room with a purse in hand, which I normally didn't carry. It would be *so* clear to these men if I headed off to the ladies room with a purse, which I didn't usually bring into the work environment. Total embarrassment! I only carried a briefcase, and I *surely* wasn't going to lug *that* into the ladies room several times a day for monthly needs! I finally figured it out after a couple of months. I would head to the ladies room just before lunch time. And, they would think I was going to lunch. Sometimes that meant I went to lunch early. I don't think men realize just *how* much thought goes into these womanly things. With the onset of menopause however, women can *finally* gain the physical freedom and mental liberation from preoccupation and worry about the reproductive cycle and all of its needs and inconveniences.

A menopausal woman will also **gain physical freedom from birth control needs, concerns, and expenses**. Menopause is the point at which a woman has not had a period for twelve consecutive months. After this point, she no longer requires birth control. So…even though a woman loses the physical ability to procreate (loss #1), she now gains the physical freedom from birth control, i.e. whether or not to utilize surgical birth control (vasectomy for him or tubal ligation for her), and she can finally say farewell to birth control products and devices for the rest of her life. No more pills, gels, foams, diaphragms, rings, shots, patches, condoms, or awkward and sometimes painful withdrawal. And, look at all the money saved. Freedom from birth control actually becomes a fantastic plus for men too, especially if he was using condoms as a form of birth control. The majority of men hate them.

With the conclusion of the reproductive years, in the fourteenth gain a woman will **gain psychological liberation, mental space, and peace of mind by not having to tend to, think about, or worry about birth control needs, concerns, nuisances, or expenses anymore**. How many times has birth control concerns thwarted a once romantic moment? A woman can now stop worrying about unwanted pregnancy and she no longer needs to think about all of the needs associated with birth control methods.

Appearing next on the list of gains, **a woman will feel rejuvenated and better overall physically and mentally after menopause**. So…even though a woman may experience a temporary loss of physical well being and/or a decreased quality of life (loss #19) while experiencing perimenopause, once she reaches menopause, she can put all of the negative perimenopausal signs, concerns, distresses, and discomforts behind her and start to feel an improvement in her physical and psychological health. I've had a few women tell me that they weighed the most they ever weighed, been the most depressed they had ever been, and felt physically worse than they had ever felt while they were in their mid-to-late forties—hormonal fluctuations and declines probably being the cause. Once hormones reach another balance after menopause however, physiological stability returns and things seem to settle down. There appears to be fewer to almost no cravings for certain foods, fewer to no monthly weight gains/losses, fewer to no monthly mood fluctuations, and PMS and similar discomforts totally disappear. It is not surprising that a woman will feel better without all of the monthly variations.

I have not experienced the rejuvenation that appears after menopause since I haven't actually reached menopause yet. But, I am truly looking forward to it. I still have some joint aches but, they don't seem as bad as when they initially emerged. And, the debilitating headaches I once experienced have started to taper off in quantity and intensity. I am not as down in the dumps as I was a year or so ago. And, I must say that so far I *have* experienced an enormous psychological development in knowledge, maturation, and spirituality.

Lastly, this feeling of overall well being was validated in a study conducted in England. According to the BBC news, the Jubilee study explored the lifestyles of women over age fifty and found that 65% of the respondents reported being happier than before menopause. Seventy-six percent of the post-menopausal women in the study stated their overall health was better, 75% stated they were having more fun, 59% stated their relationships improved, and 93% stated they felt they had more independence and more choice in everything from work to leisure pursuits.[147]

Appearing last on the list of gains as number sixteen, a woman will **gain a certain confidence and self-assurance after perimenopause**. (1) As the outcome of a life experience that has reached the approximate half-way point, i.e. from invaluable lessons learned in the life experience, (2) from the self-evaluation and life inventory that has occurred during this time of life, (3) from the personal development in decision-making ability, (4) from the priority assessment and/or priority shifting, and (5) from the management of perimenopause itself, a woman is probably *more* aware now than ever before of what she wants, what makes her happy, and where she wants to go. She has probably learned how to manage her emotions better through all of the perimenopausal turmoil and added responsibilities of mid-life, she is probably more in touch with her own feelings, and she is probably more comfortable in her physical being, i.e. she's grown into herself. So...even though a perimenopausal woman may initially have faced identity loss and/or role confusion (loss #2), a loss of/or a change in a caring attitude (loss #10), and/or a loss of body and/or self image (loss #16), she will most likely emerge from the entire perimenopause process having *totally* redefined herself and feeling more comfortable and content than ever before. I actually started seeing and feeling this newfound confidence approximately one year after I started experiencing perimenopausal signs—it was definitely a process though.

This new, self-assured demeanor that emerges in the perimenopausal woman reminds me of an employee in the workplace, one who has experience and seniority, and one who has had *many, many* years on the job. This distinguished employee exudes a certain poise and self-confidence that reflects her extensive experience level. There is a particular knowledge, skill, and ability base and "seasoning" this experienced employee brings to the table that is evident in her demeanor. And, she is especially respected and valued by others in the workplace. Similarly, a woman who has reached perimenopause becomes "seasoned" in the life experience—her overall knowledge, life skills, and accumulated abilities ascend to another level in this place called life.

In review, the **gains/benefits of perimenopause, menopause, and post menopause** are:

1. Gain an understanding or gain specific knowledge of future goals, aspirations, and objectives through reflection on the past

2. Gain awareness that life has reached the approximate half-way mark—time element suddenly becomes important

3. Experience a priority assessment and/or a priority shift

4. Gain entrance into a huge milestone in the lifespan

5. Gain the advantage of being totally tuned into the physical being

6. Gain the knowledge that there is control managing perimenopause via a variety of options

7. Newfound respect and admiration for mother, other female family members, or female friends and potential improvement in these relationships

8. Gain new relationships during perimenopause

9. Gain extra time, flexibility, and/or money

10. Gain mental space and peace of mind in relation to family planning

11. Gain the physical freedom from a monthly cycle

12. Gain psychological liberation, mental space, and peace of mind from tending to, thinking about, and worrying about monthly needs, concerns, nuisances, aches, pains, and expenses

13. Gain physical freedom from birth control needs, concerns, and expenses

14. Gain psychological liberation, mental space, and peace of mind from tending to, thinking about, and worrying about birth control needs, concerns, nuisances, and expenses

15. Rejuvenation/feeling better overall physically and mentally after menopause

16. Gain a certain confidence and self-assurance

# 5

# *Perimenopause and Other Significant Life Events*

Perimenopause is another life experience, like adolescence or aging. Unfortunately, the onset of perimenopause happens at a time in a woman's life when other major, external life-altering events are most likely also taking place (these events affect men too). It is not enough to have to deal with the many personal physical and psychological issues that may transpire during perimenopause, but a woman must *also* confront other external matters that can crop up during this time. These additional life circumstances can easily force alterations in social roles, job or career requirements, financial stability, and/or living arrangements. The perimenopausal woman may find herself stretching her adaptation resources to the limit to assimilate and accommodate all of the different things that she is now faced with.[148] Additionally, these peripheral concerns may contribute to increasing her stress levels and can complicate life even further for her making perimenopause seem like an extra burden that has to be "dealt with". It should be mentioned that men can also experience some of these same important mid-life events, except that they are not confronting perimenopause with all of its concerns, issues, demands, and stresses at the same time.

Some significant life-changing situations that can occur concurrently with perimenopause include, but are not limited to the following:

1. **Full nest**: Since an increasing number of women are starting families well into their forties, a woman may have the added responsibilities of a new **baby or even babies** which can undoubtedly increase stress levels during perimenopause. In fact, one in five women today (worldwide) are waiting to start families after the age of thirty-five.[149]

2. **Full nest including an adolescent**: It should be mentioned that a child in or entering the teenage years can be *extremely* taxing for any parent, much less a perimenopausal woman. My twelve year old son was demanding, verbally experimental, argumentative, stubborn, and totally self-absorbed, as countless teenagers are. He posed many new challenges for me on a daily basis that only added to the pressures of perimenopause.

3. **Empty nest syndrome**: Empty nest syndrome refers to the grief that parents may experience upon their child or children leaving home.[150] Women, in general, experience empty nest syndrome more often and more intensely than men. This is understandable since they have probably been the parent most plugged into the child as the primary care giver.[151] A woman's life will change suddenly one day when her child leaves home and the daily caretaking duties of being a mother that once determined her lifestyle are no longer needed in the child's absence. The child may have left the home to attend college, to get married, to become independent in this great big world, or to establish some other living arrangement. Whatever the reason for the child leaving, it does not seem to lessen the grief in empty nest syndrome. Of course, a mother is a mother forever, but the main hands-on tasks of motherhood are not necessary any longer once the child has moved out. And, a woman's life minus her child now becomes *extremely* altered from the way it was before, especially if the child pretty much dictated her lifestyle. Some women actually lose their sense of purpose in life once the child leaves.

Along with all of the sadness, emptiness, isolation, and other emotions of missing a child's daily presence in the home, this is actually a *very* positive event in a woman's life psychologically. It is another *huge* milestone in the lifespan. A woman who has successfully reared a child can now kick back with feelings of intense relief, pride, and satisfaction that she has raised an independent, productive, and valuable member of society.

4. **New family members**: Many women in our society today are postponing having a family until later in life for various reasons (delaying commitment/marriage, financial concerns, career aspirations/demands, etc.). A woman may very well be entering perimenopause with a small infant/child in the home. This may also be a time when new significant others and/or new in-laws are introduced into the family and/or a grandchild/grandchildren come into the world. These new relationships in turn are responsible for social role adjustments for the perimenopausal woman.

5. **Aging/Ill parent(s)**: An aging parent(s) with deteriorating physical and/or mental health may require extra care and attention at this time. Any additional time that has been gained from an empty nest may have to be utilized caring for an aging and/or ill parent(s) Even if the perimenopausal woman does not physically care for the elderly/ill parent(s) in her home, nursing home placement or any out-placement for that matter has its own unique set of complicated decisions and challenges: (1) Where should the parent(s) go? With the perimenopausal woman? With her siblings? Or, with other family members who could be located in another state or even another country. Or, would the parent(s) be better off in an assisted living facility or a nursing home? (2) If the parent(s) does go to a living facility, what sort of facility can the parent(s) afford? (3) Once the parent(s) has been placed in the facility, who will manage the parent(s) money, property, and/or other assets? Can this designated person be trusted to handle this task responsibly? These are just a few of the concerns that can materialize in regard to an aging/ill parent(s) welfare which can easily force major responsibilities/decisions/emotional turmoil on the perimenopausal woman.

Also, as the perimenopausal woman observes her own parent(s) face his/her own mortality, this may create more stresses, tensions, and/or anxieties as she herself considers and faces her own aging and finiteness upon approaching middle age. As I write this book, my own mother recently turned 86. She has had a total knee replacement, a vascular stent insertion, a fractured vertebra, and a partial shoulder surgery in a matter of a year!

6. **Loss of a parent(s)**: This may be a time when an elderly or ill parent passes on which may be devastating for the perimenopausal woman. And, if one parent is left behind, this too, can create added responsibilities for the perimenopausal woman, especially if the existing parent is in ill or deteriorating health and requires extra time and/or attention.

7. **Aging/Ill/Loss of a pet(s)**: This may be a time when a family pet(s) becomes ill or even passes on. As another member of the family, this may impose emotional mayhem, and/or added responsibilities/time obligations/additional expenses on the perimenopausal woman with vet visits, medication purchases, medication administration, and other necessary requirements/treatments for an aging/ill pet(s). More importantly the emotionality of coping with a cherished pet's illness or even death can be overwhelming for the perimenopausal woman who may already be in an emotionally charged state.

8. **Split/Separation/Divorce**: Due to various circumstances, the time of peri-menopause may be a time when a relationship split, separation, or divorce happens or even seems like the best option. For example, if a child has recently left home, and the couple remained together in a poor relationship/marriage for the sake of the child, there really is no reason to continue to stay together and the couple may now decide to end the relationship. This situation alone can easily thrust a woman into many different directions: emotionally, physically, financially, etc. Statistically, a woman's standard of living generally decreases with a divorce, which adds a whole new set of worries. With the loss of a significant other's/spouse's income, she may find herself requiring additional financial earnings. This may force her into having to search for new employment, or if she is already employed, she may have to increase her work hours to make ends meet. This is not as simple as it sounds, because the older one gets, the more difficult it becomes to integrate into the workforce from both ends, i.e. from the employee's perspective and also from the employer's perspective. Furthermore, if the peri-menopausal woman requires additional education and/or skills to locate a decent job, she may find herself back in school in middle age.

Not only can relationship breakdowns, financial pressures, and job pressures wreak havoc in her life, but social roles may change for her as well. More often than not accompanying a split/separation/divorce comes social role adjustments. She may lose current friends, neighbors, work peers, and/or in-laws and gain new friends, neighbors, work peers and/or in-laws. And, of course, a split/separation/divorce may lead to another new close/intimate relationship. Also, if the peri-menopausal woman finds herself working extremely long hours to make ends meet, she my have *little* to *no* social interaction at all.

Finally, a relationship split/separation/divorce coinciding with perimenopause may leave a woman feeling lonely, abandoned, isolated, and/or depressed at a time when she really needs the emotional support from a significant other/spouse. Divorce, separation, or any other relationship split and the emotional, physical, employment, and financial pressures that can ensue may come at a *most* inopportune time as a woman tries to contend with her own set of issues in peri-menopause.

9. **Illness/Loss of a significant other/Spouse**: A significant other or a spouse may become ill or even pass on. This can be a serious hardship emotionally as well as a financial hardship for the perimenopausal woman. Emotionally, if she is already down in the dumps from being in a perimenopausal state, the illness or loss of a significant other/spouse will only compound her depression. She may

find herself single again in her fifties, when dating and reintroducing herself back into society may not come as easily as it once did. Or, she may find herself out in the workforce again trying to make ends meet. Or, she may find herself in a serious financial bind due to the significant other's/spouse's illness or death.

**10. Residence change (Downsize/Expansion):** Many times when a child leaves the home, less dwelling space becomes necessary and the perimenopausal woman (and her significant other) may decide to downsize an existing home. Or, on the other hand, with the birth of a new baby(s), and/or adding new in-laws, and/or adding elderly/ill family members to the home, *more* living space may be needed. Along with all the downscaling/upscaling that may be happening, there will be a loss of a previous lifestyle. Moving is right up there on top of the stress scale too.

**11. Career pressures/Demands/Changes:** Perimenopause can become a time when a career change is considered, sometimes not necessarily voluntarily. Unfortunately, life occasionally throws a curve ball that forces a change of career and sometimes at the most inconvenient times, like in the midst of perimenopause! Which…may be the *worst* time for a career move! However, keep in mind that most of the changes we experience in the life experience *are* somewhat forced. Most of us will *not* actively seek change if things are status quo.

For me, I had a great job with an aircraft manufacturer when I suddenly found myself (along with 149 others) unemployed one February day. This was the second time I had been laid off from the same company and it really turned my life upside down this time. I did *not* want to settle for another job and take a large pay decrease because we couldn't afford for me to do that. And, with a sagging economy, there weren't many jobs out there anyway. Sadly, with little money coming into the household, an adolescent son, and me going through perimenopause, I just didn't have a clue how I would make it through day-to-day. All I could do was to take life one day at a time. I kept trying to figure out the lesson I was supposed to be learning in these lean times. I *had* always wanted to author a book and decided while I was looking for the right job, I would start writing this book. I *threw* myself into this project and as difficult as it became financially, I was so *very* happy writing!!! I knew that I had finally found the *perfect* job for me. It was my passion that I was finally able to pursue.

As mentioned previously, if the perimenopausal woman has split/separated/divorced/lost her significant other/spouse and she now discovers that she needs additional income, she may find herself back in school, changing careers (to increase her earning potential), or pursuing a new career outside the home (if she stayed at home). This may add *extreme* pressure and demands on the perimenopausal woman to be able to earn a comparable amount of money (as in the relationship) to maintain a certain lifestyle.

Furthermore, in a world of frequent and now so common corporate restructures, mergers, takeovers, and downsizes, there may be *many* more demands and responsibilities placed on employees in the workplace than ever before. For example, many organizations are now requiring that their employees be cross-trained, in other words do the job of *many* people. And, if a downsizing occurs (remember that I have been through two of these myself), existing employees may automatically end up performing many additional duties of the employees who are gone. The current corporate environment can *certainly* add numerous pressures, demands, and responsibilities on the perimenopausal woman.

12. **Financial concerns**: There are many factors that can contribute to financial shifts during this time of life. There may be career changes (forced or elective), there may be relationship issues, i.e. split/separation/divorce/illness/death, there may be parental issues, i.e. illness/loss of independence/death, retirement, illness, or a multitude of other issues that can impose financial pressures, demands, and/ or changes on the perimenopausal woman.

13. **Retirement**: Perimenopause may be a time when a woman (or her significant other/spouse) may be retiring from the workforce permanently, or at least considering retirement. It seems the closer I came to retirement, the more it and all of its financial constraints and concerns plagued me. *How much money would I need? How many years after retirement would I need money? Would Social Security even be around when I retired?* There were so many unknowns.

Retirement may be a time of financial concerns, but it can also force social role changes on the perimenopausal woman. For instance, work peers and/or friends may be lost while other friends may be found.

# 6

# *Perimenopausal Issues*

*How long are these things that are happening to me going to last? What am I going to look like when this is over? What am I going to be like when this is over?* These are only a few of the questions that popped into my mind frequently nowadays. And in fact, at times, it seemed as if perimenopause with all of its issues and concerns was consuming a great deal of my mental energy. Upon researching for this book, I realized that there are actually several different issues that may surface at various times during the perimenopause phase. Some of these issues are triggered by perimenopause itself and other issues occur due to the parallel time frame of perimenopause with mid-life. The inconsistent nature of perimenopause *within* each woman and the differences *between* women may also trigger other issues. This chapter investigates these perimenopausal issues further. (Please note that a few of the issues mentioned in this chapter may overlap other areas of the book, but I felt it was necessary to identify them as perimenopausal issues and to expound on them even further.)

## 1. Perimenopause is continuously in the back of the mind:

*Why do I have to go through this?* I initially wondered, dreading the inevitable.

Now that I acknowledged the ramifications of middle-age, **perimenopause was *continuously* in the back of my mind**. I couldn't seem to shake it. With every ache and pain I experienced, with every unrestful night I struggled through, and with every impatient moment I found myself in, I wondered if perimenopause was to blame. It seemed as if it was always right there in the back of my mind all the time. One woman, who had already experienced menopause, advised me that if there were only a few things in the course of the day that bothered me, it was probably those few things that were truly bothersome. But…if *everything* in the course of the day bothered me, which seemed to be happening frequently nowadays, then it was definitely my hormones. From the negative perimenopausal signs that I had recently been experiencing, the joint aches, irritability, mood swings, and cognitive changes, I knew that I had entered into the perimenopause progression. It was difficult *not* to think about it!

## 2. The time of perimenopause is a milestone/midlife marker:

Psychologically and chronologically speaking, **perimenopause is a *very* significant milestone** in a woman's life, as mentioned earlier. It is an approximate **midlife marker** in a woman's lifespan. Physically speaking, there are the major hormonal shifts that will affect a woman's existence, just as menarche marked the beginning of, and influenced her childbearing years. How each woman mentally perceives and receives perimenopause is totally individualistic, similar to the perceptual differences in the beginning of the childbearing years. Much of the overall perception of perimenopause, and how a woman enters and experiences the process, has to do with her previous exposure to, education, and experience with the topic. Some women will perceive perimenopause as a sign of aging and are truly *horrified* at reaching this midlife marker, while other women will perceive perimenopause as a new beginning in the lifespan, graciously accepting and embracing it. Some women will miss the attractiveness of younger years. And, some women will associate perimenopause and the aging process with unattractiveness and distastefulness. On the other hand, some women are willing and prepared to accept maturation, viewing the perimenopause process as a positive passage in the life cycle. These women look forward to the freedom, independence, and growth that ultimately accompany menopause. Some women may also fear losing their fertility, associating it with a loss of femininity and/or a loss of womanhood, while other women may gladly relinquish their childbearing years as they anticipate a new-found freedom. Regardless of how each woman identifies perimenopause, it still signifies a mid-life marker.

## 3. Mid-life assessment occurs now:

Another issue that will surface during perimenopause is a mental **mid-life evaluation**. Do you remember hearing about how some mid-lifers would experience a "mid-life crisis"? In an attempt to feel young again they might impulsively run out and purchase something that might make them feel younger. Something like a bright, cherry red corvette. Well, this is it, the mid-life transition. This is the time when we (women and men alike) evaluate our lives up to this point. We tend to focus inward, thoughtfully reviewing our achievements, struggles, failures, relationships, careers, health, etc. At first, I was not aware that a mid-life evaluation was even taking place. I would find myself on occasion mentally reviewing past life choices and their outcomes until reflective and evaluative thoughts started popping into my head more and more frequently, at times bombarding me, and that's when I finally become cognizant of the fact that I was in a mid-life evaluation.

Typically, an individual will also assess lifetime **successes and accomplishments** in mid-life. There are many wonderful things that have happened in each and every one of our lives. And, we need to feel confident that some of the decisions we made and the goals we achieved were indeed accomplishments and successes. It is important that we feel a sense of pride and satisfaction in them. (This especially becomes important toward the end of the lifespan.)

In our society, these successes/failures are most likely measured by:

1. the quality of interpersonal relationships

2. educational level

3. occupation

4. financial status

5. social status

Furthermore, new challenges may accompany the mid-life experience. A woman may find herself facing a whole new set of unique and demanding roles as mentioned earlier, i.e. caring for aging/ill parents, a child/children leaving home, an aging/ill family pet, new grandchildren, new in-laws, or she may find herself facing new life challenges such as relocation, new job, retirement, downsizing, unemployment, etc. As for myself, there seemed to be a new challenge on a daily basis during this perimenopausal phase! Adversity was something I was becoming very used to and almost comfortable with.

Finally, as a result of the mid-life evaluation, most individuals will emerge with a **new self impression**. It is very interesting how some people perceive their own successes/failures. One person may consider another individual as *very* successful and financially stable, say for example, a Vice-President of a major corporation earning seven figures annually plus bonuses and other perks. Yet, in actuality that very same Vice-President is really quite frustrated and very depressed; he does not feel successful in life because he isn't the *President* of the corporation and he isn't making more money to have acquired more stuff.

## 4. We are reminded of own physical finiteness/mortality now:

We women may **frequently be reminded of our own physical finiteness** with the many aches and pains that accompany perimenopause and we may become *very* aware of our own mortality now. When we have a simple cut that now takes *weeks* to heal instead of the mere days it took to heal in more youthful days, we are brutally made aware of the aging process and ultimately our own mortality. If we have aging or ill parents/significant others/spouses/other family members/ friends and/or pets, we may also become painfully aware of own mortality as we watch them face their own aging, illness, or even death.

It's funny, because when most of us realize that we really *are* middle-aged, it is with much disbelief and trepidation and not with satisfaction and pleasure.[152] Instead of feeling a sense of pride and achievement about having made it this far in life, most of us cringe at the thought of mid-life and moving forward from here. Instead of being thankful for becoming invested in this tangible experience we call life, we are unappreciative and feel deprived of infinite youth. I have actually heard some individuals refer to the aging process as "punishment on earth". Certain people I have spoken with felt that by living and consequently aging, and having to experience all the aches and pains of aging, that they were somehow being penalized. Dying seems to be an easier alternative than life for some people.

## 5. Unknown fear factors: (1) Perimenopausal signs, (2) Final body type:

Another concern in perimenopause has to do with **unknown fear factors**. There are two major fears in particular during perimenopause that I have identified. (1) The **unexpectedness and inconsistency in occurrence of perimenopausal signs** may leave a woman wondering whether the signs will last for three hours, three days, or three years! This is extremely *frightening* for a woman when she has no idea when, where, to what degree, or for how long any of the perimenopausal signs will last. If, for instance, a woman experiences hot flashes on two successive nights, she has no clue when they will disappear, reappear, or if she will be spending another week, another year, or even worse yet, years with them. The cerebral aspect of *not* knowing what will happen, for how long it will happen, or when it will happen, is fear-provoking for any woman. The unknown and the unfamiliar are typically scary to humans, as I mentioned earlier (except for maybe the few risk-takers who thrive on the unknown). In middle-age, we have grown rather comfortable with the familiar aspects of life. We have settled into our own bodies, our surroundings, and our routines. We may not respond as enthusiastically or as quickly to new and different things, especially when they interfere with daily existence as we know it.

Another unknown fear factor in perimenopause is (2) the **fear of *not* knowing what the "more mature" body shape will eventually look like**. Even with plenty of exercise and proper nutrition, there is still some "settling in", or physical redistribution that occurs during this time. Many women notice an abdominal "pooch" or thickening and/or a fat redistribution or change in composition. Some women may actually lose weight during this time of life, especially with all of the stress of other significant life events that may be occurring simultaneously with perimenopause. But, generally speaking, most women will gain a few pounds. So…it is quite understandable for a woman to wonder what her physical appearance will morph into.

## 6. Perimenopause occurs in the company of the aging process, making it difficult to separate the two:

**The aging process itself is occurring at the same time as perimenopause**. It becomes difficult to identify exactly when perimenopause, with its hormonal fluctuations and declines, kicks in and/or when the aging process alone is responsible for signs of aging. Perimenopause takes place at a time in life when the aging process is also beginning to take hold of the individual and its presence is becoming noticeable to a certain degree. And, since some women experience perimenopause for years, it becomes *really* tricky trying to tease out the aging process from the perimenopause process. Furthermore, given that men also experience the same signs of aging as women (sensory changes, skin changes, hair loss, weight gain, etc.) female hormonal fluctuations and declines alone *cannot* solely be responsible for all of the changes that a woman undergoes during perimenopause.

# 7

# *Why Such a Bad Rap?:*
# *Why Aren't Women Talking*
# *About Perimenopause?*

Women are actually doing more harm to themselves than good by *not* openly discussing perimenopause. It has been suggested that a failure to express personal thoughts and feelings can lead to a sense of isolation, a loss of/or a distorted perspective, and/or an increase in concerns and anxiety. I certainly felt very isolated in this life experience. Women may also be capturing a skewed picture of the perimenopause process by only picking up bits and pieces here and there from various sources, indeed not a complete and accurate depiction of the process. There are many explanations why women are not communicating freely, i.e. talking, sharing, inquiring, and listening about perimenopause. And, it is really not too hard to understand *why* the entire menopause transition has received such lukewarm reception, resulting in this huge communication gap, if we simply review some of the facts below:

First and foremost, the **menopause process was, and still remains an accepted part of the medical model** in our society. Being part of this paradigm implies that a disease process or medical condition is occurring. Historically, menopause was considered a "hormone deficiency" that needed some medical treatment and/or some sort of medical intervention. In the early 1950's for example, menopause was actually recognized as an "estrogen deficiency" disease. This particular assessment, diagnosis, and treatment plan *easily* creates the expectation that a woman will probably be experiencing negative signs during perimenopause and will, no doubt, need some sort of therapeutic treatment or medicinal intervention (most likely HT) for the rest of her life. Having a background in the medical field myself and having a few personal experiences with medicine (birth of my son, etc.), I would like to mention that I am *not* against the medical model. There are many wonderful doctors, treatments, medicines, and procedures available today. However, the way the menopause transition has been viewed and treated *in* the medical model has, in my opinion, been a negative force on women.

Subsequently, another notable dark cloud that has continued to negatively affect the general public's perception of menopause is that it has been established as a medical condition in the medical model for *half* the population (women) that **requires some sort of pharmacologic treatment** for thirty or more years in a woman's lifetime.[153] What are the implications of that? However, in light of recent HT findings, which indicated that in many cases the risks outweighed the benefits, there has been a shift in thinking. Due to the possible harmful side effects of HT, other medical treatments must now be established and utilized in treating negative perimenopausal signs. Maybe this shift in thinking will result in a return to more natural methods in treating negative perimenopausal signs.

Furthermore, the menopause transition is portrayed as **a physical disorder** that will undoubtedly trigger other health problems. It is true that there can be some temporary discomforts and inconveniences during the perimenopause process, but these are mostly short-lived and a state of well health/homeostasis☺ is eventually restored. And, even though there is a decline in hormone levels, they do eventually equalize (in lesser amounts) as they are produced in other parts of the body; the adrenal glands, the liver, the kidneys and fat cells aid in estrogen conversion, for example. Additionally, a diet rich in calcium and/or calcium supplements can help prevent or delay osteoporosis before, during, and after menopause. A woman's eating habits, exercise routine, living environment, financial status, social status, genetics, medical condition, and history of these just mentioned items are also extremely important to her general wellness. Declines in hormone levels during perimenopause cannot be blamed for *all* ill health. For example, if a woman has been an overweight smoker, who rarely exercised most of her life, and who lives in an urban or industrialized neighborhood exposing her to poor air quality, toxic chemicals, noise pollution, etc., then she cannot rightfully blame her heart attack on estrogen loss!

Additionally, women who once sought medical attention for perimenopausal signs probably did so because of (1) **a *pervasive* lack of open communication about perimenopause**, (2) **a lack of emotional support from loved ones and friends, and** (3) **a lack of other female role models**.[154] In the past, this severe gap in menopausal communication, the limited information available, and limited access to the information left many women with no other choice *but* to seek help and information from a health care provider.

Following the above mentioned communication gap, another reason why menopause may have developed negatively in our society is the fact that because people didn't openly discuss it, **the silence that surrounded the process resulted in society perceiving it as a frightening event and in the worst terms possible**. There was never any other open communication or indication to suggest otherwise.

Another inaccurate perception of menopause is this **culture's general adaptation of the experience**. Taking a look back in time can explain how this dismal adaptation came to be. Historically, the human lifespan was much shorter than it is today. In fact, the human life expectancy was only fifty years of age in the 19th century.[155] Old age and even death was not far behind menopause, which was considered a precursor to death, which it was! And, similar to the subject of death in those times, communication about menopause was considered a taboo subject and any open discussion about the process was mostly discouraged. Menopause, therefore, developed into a life event that was silenced—people just didn't talk about it. Unfortunately, cultural traditions and mores continue on even after they no longer apply. For that very reason it could take *years* for menopause to become an event that is accepted, honored, and openly discussed in our society.

Given that the overall perception and experience of the menopause process is so culturally dependent, let's look at some universal differences in a more positive light. In India, for example, the women in a few prominent social castes experience hardly *any* negative perimenopausal signs. These women enthusiastically anticipate menopause in their lives as there are many social rewards associated with this life event.[156] They are revered and considered valued members of their society with the passage of menopause with the knowledge and wisdom that life has brought them. These women maintain the same important work functions after menopause and are now able to socialize with males (other than their husbands) and frequent places they once before did not or could not visit.[157]

Japanese women don't experience many of the negative signs that American women confront in perimenopause. They don't even have a term for hot flashes! It has been suggested that Japanese diets are supplemented most of their lives with foods that contain very high levels of natural estrogens, mainly soy products. Therefore, it is theorized that this particular diet provides natural estrogen supplementation continuously throughout their lives so that when the menopause transition finally does arrive, there are enough hormones present allowing the body to substitute and divert any negative perimenopausal signs. Furthermore, these women *seldom* get breast cancer. It has also been asserted that this particular culture may actually discourage verbal expression of complaints about negative signs of perimenopause. Another interesting fact is that Japanese women have the world's longest life expectancy of 85.2 years (2002).[158] Could there be a correlation between diet, cultural attitudes, cultural expectations and the menopause transition and life expectancy?

Likewise, Chinese women report no major negative perimenopausal signs. Interestingly, cultures such as the ones just mentioned (India, Japan, China) that celebrate and honor menopause and have positive attitudes and expectations about the aging process[159] appear to have a decreased incidence of negative perimenopausal signs.

The National Institutes of Health (NIH)☺ expounds on the premise that in this culture **menopause has been perceived mainly in negative terms** as a life transition dominated by distressing physical and psychological signs.[160] According to the NIH, the documentation of occurrence of negative perimenopausal signs could have in fact been the result of an **over-sampling of clinical populations seeking treatment for perimenopausal signs** and not a true measurement of occurrence of negative perimenopausal signs in the general population.

Many women may also be reluctant discussing perimenopause because of the **overall misinformation and unfortunate expectations that still exist**. As mentioned earlier, in Western societies there is a medical nature that has been attached to the entire menopause process. Perimenopausal women in this culture may feel that they are ill to some degree and they really don't want to/or are embarrassed to discuss their alleged medical problems with anyone else. And, since perimenopause is considered such a marked age delineation separating middle adulthood from the older, more mature population, women may also feel hesitant to publicly admit to and enter into that world of maturity. Remember, we live in a culture where youth dominates many facets of our daily existence and we attempt to fit in with that population for as long as possible.

Additionally, some perimenopausal women are not talking because the **perimenopausal signs they may be experiencing are so subtle and gradual, they may have no idea that they are even in perimenopause**. My own perimenopause first surfaced as vague, intermittent joint pain. Who would have guessed that perimenopause was actually inching its way into my life manifesting itself as stiff and achy joints? How can a woman even talk about perimenopause when she is unaware of its existence? This is exactly what the BBC reported from a recent survey that found half of British women cope with perimenopausal signs for at least a *year* without recognizing that perimenopause has arrived. Also according to the BBC, a survey by The Choices Campaign, conducted by the HRT Aware

Group, found that one in four women do not even recognize perimenopausal signs for up the three years![161]

Some women may feel that perimenopause is a **private matter** and they simply aren't comfortable disclosing such personal information to others. Many individuals (different generations, for example) may have been raised to feel that these matters were personal and best kept private. For instance, my mother, who is in her eighties, and her cohorts certainly kept such information confidential and any related discussion was kept under wraps. And, who raised people like me? People of that generation, that is, people who didn't discuss these matters openly or candidly.

The Baby Boom generation on the other hand (of which I am one), seems to be *much* freer in its expression and much more conscientious in its information seeking endeavors than its parents' generation with regard to menopause and the mid-life experience. Having myself been part of the "Sexual Revolution", I would agree that sex and associated topics are probably discussed more openly today by Boomers. However, from *my* experience with other women of all ages including many Boomers, it seems that there still remains plenty of reluctance and caution when talking about perimenopause. And, even though a cohort effect exists as I stated above (more open, less open, etc.), the way each individual was raised is very important in what is communicated and how it is communicated.

**Embarrassment** may be another reason why women are uncomfortable communicating about perimenopause. This issue includes the following considerations: **First**, some individuals find it awkward discussing *any* sexually related topic with someone else including a sexual partner. **Second**, many women in our society are *extremely* uncomfortable discussing their age, or age-related issues, which is probably typical in a culture where a more youthful orientation prevails. And, as already clearly established, perimenopause implies that middle-age has arrived. **Third**, the perimenopausal woman may also feel a sense of humility in disclosing delicate information about herself to others. **Fourth**, if she does open up exposing herself to others, they may casually dismiss her concerns offering her absolutely no emotional support (which is what she may have been looking for), which in turn may leave her feeling sorry and/or embarrassed that she ever shared her thoughts and emotions with anyone at all.

Women may also fail to be communicating to others about perimenopause because of feelings of **personal mismanagement**. A woman may feel or believe that it is solely *her* responsibility to manage her own body, hence her own perimenopause. By admitting to or discussing any perimenopausal concerns or signs that she may be experiencing, she might perhaps believe that she has been unsuccessful or even consider herself a failure in the handling of her own personal matters.

Because women are *not* talking about perimenopause with each other and apparently not with their doctors, they may be **missing out on valuable and useful information** that could help them better acknowledge and assimilate this mid-life event. The media does offer some health information, but women may not be getting all the facts they need when it comes to perimenopause. They may only be getting informational fragments here and there and not the complete picture. It really would benefit women to open up, talk about, and elicit information from each other about this mid-life event, because as indicated earlier, sharing stories and other specifics is an invaluable way to gather valuable and useful information in the life experience.

# 8

# *Triumph: Mental Management Strategies*

Now that we have a good handle on perimenopause and its many complex aspects and associated issues, i.e. (1) the physiological changes, (2) the psychological changes, (3) the losses, (4) the grieving, (5) other significant life events, (6) the issues, and (7) the lack of communication, let's explore some of the ways a woman can mentally meet and triumph over the negative affects of this major and inevitable life event. How can a woman decrease her chances of experiencing negative signs during perimenopause? What sorts of things can she do to cope with the negative aspects of perimenopause? And…how can she enter into this stage of life with a healthy, optimistic attitude? What can the perimenopausal woman do to overcome the pessimistic consciousness surrounding the menopause transition that currently exists in our culture?

*Every* woman should start her **perimenopause management protocol** with some sort of education and then employ a combination of other strategies that are mentioned below. This will (1) empower her, (2) help guide her through the process, (3) help reduce negative perimenopausal signs, (4) positively impact her outward appearance and inward perspective, and (5) help her feel better overall. Read on.

## 1. Educate:

Once again, the importance of being informed and knowledgeable cannot be emphasized enough. **Education** is *instrumental* in arriving at this place in life with any amount of preparation, confidence, and enthusiasm. Education helps a woman navigate through this time of many changes in several ways. She will: (1) learn about the physical and psychological **nature of hormonal shifts** and the implications of such fluctuations and declines, (2) learn about the many **losses and gains** she may experience, (3) learn about the many **options** available to her in treating the signs of perimenopause, and (4) learn how to **manage her emotions**. Furthermore, a woman will discover that she is only one of the millions upon millions of women who are **morphing or who have already morphed through the same thing**. I found that the more I researched the subject, the more empowered I felt because I then knew exactly what to expect. Even though there are differences between women, the general passage through perimenopause is the same. And, by uncovering the mystery and removing inaccuracies about perimenopause, a woman will become more knowledgeable and consequently better equipped to deal with the process. Let's face it, knowledge is power. And, if a woman can equip herself with *all* of the educational tools she can gather, she can easily address and manage her own personal perimenopause from its onset. As a final point on the topic of education, a woman should *keep* herself informed, even after the initial information gathering stage, as information seems to change on an almost daily basis.

Most recently, with the increasing female Baby Boomer population reaching mid-life, there seems to be a "do-it-yourself" trend in the direction of investigating the menopause transition. The availability and easier accessibility (via new technology) to accurate information in this information age has made research much less difficult and less time consuming than in the past. Even though women still seem somewhat hesitant to speak openly about their own personal perimenopause, as was my experience, they *are* seeking informative material from medical and non-medical sources alike to help them through the process. So women *are* beginning to become informed and they are staying informed.

## 2. Don't fear perimenopause because it's a natural, biological process:

From what I had been exposed to about the menopause process in general, I understood it to be a very negative and frightening experience that catapulted a woman into old age! I really didn't know what to expect, especially with most of the people I knew being so reluctant to talk about it. But, as I researched the topic, I came to realize that perimenopause, and ultimately menopause, was certainly nothing to be fearful of at all. It was *not* some sort of affliction or disease as the medical model so strongly suggests. It was *not* some phenomenon that thrust a woman into old age. It was merely a natural biological occurrence, like any other life experience, that was going to transpire regardless. And as I have already stated, the more I learned about it, the less I dreaded it.

If you think about it, *every* living thing on this earth seems to have a natural integrated circuitry built into it that programs the organism, keeping it on a particular track. We humans experience life pretty much at the same pace. As babies, we roll over at approximately a few months of age, we start walking upright at about a year old, and we experience adolescence in teen years, etc. We have been physically pre-wired or encoded for certain events to take place, such as the aging process, as specified in Leonard Hayflick's (1961) "programmed theory of aging" (even though newer theories have emerged since, Hayflick's theory still holds a lot of merit). He discovered that cells have a finite lifespan and he asserted that aging is an event that transpires because it is programmed into our cells. So if we view perimenopause in that light, **it is just a natural progression that is predetermined** for us. It is a universal experience that reaches every woman on every continent. It could not be more natural.

When I was pregnant with my son, I was *petrified* of the entire childbirth experience, as I have a very low tolerance to any sort of pain or discomfort. But, I also felt that it was the most natural thing in the world. Luckily, it all worked out. My son was a breech baby (a C-section) and even though I experienced some post-op pain, I never experienced any labor or birth pain. Thank God for good doctors, epidurals, and morphine! The anticipation was really much worse than the actual event. Likewise with perimenopause, preconceptions about the process are probably much worse than the actual event.

### 3. Acknowledge perimenopause and accept it and it then becomes easier to manage:

Once a woman **recognizes that perimenopause has arrived**, and understands what is actually happening to her, she will have an easier time accepting and managing the changes. For me, once I became aware of the signs, i.e. joint stiffness, mood fluctuations, etc. and acknowledged them as part of the perimenopause process, I was better able to accept and manage them. While developing this book and at the same time educating myself about perimenopause, I became much more competent and in turn confident in anticipating and accepting the process more readily. From what my body was telling me and from what the literature was conveying to me, most of the negative perimenopausal signs would be transient anyway and they would disappear at some point (for instance, the headaches I was experiencing had already subsided and the joint aches weren't as bad). I found that the most effective way to handle the negative perimenopausal signs was to do so as they surfaced. In other words, care for the negative signs with the goal of soothing them and reducing the discomforts, until in time they would vanish. In my case, I chose not to use HT of BHRT.

Many women are *not* cognizant of the fact that they are indeed experiencing perimenopause as mentioned previously. They go about their busy and hectic daily routines really having no clue that they are entering or are already in the midst of perimenopause. Any negative, and often-times ambiguous, perimenopausal signs the woman may experience are shrugged off and/or disregarded. If a woman is not sure that she is experiencing perimenopause, a simple test can be done to ascertain that perimenopause has begun. The test works by detecting increasing levels of follicle stimulating hormone (FSH) which indicates a positive result ascertaining the woman is in perimenopause (FSH blood level greater than 50mlU/mg). The test is available through health care professionals and there is also a home version, similar to a home pregnancy test, which uses urine to activate it. Estrogen levels can also be tested to determine if perimenopause has begun. This is indicated if the estradiol serum level is less than 50pg/ml.

## 4. Meet perimenopause directly:

The fourth component in managing perimenopause effectively is for the woman to **meet the perimenopause process head-on**. Denying the fact that middle age and with it perimenopause has tiptoed into her life is going to make it more difficult for a woman to manage her perimenopause. Denial of this life event can also prevent personal growth and development from occurring. We have all, at one point or another, procrastinated or failed to confront something by putting it off only to find that once we faced it and dealt with it, it really wasn't as terrible as we thought it was going to be. If we deal with any matter directly, we can mentally move on to something else rather than have the thing hanging over our heads consuming our energies.

## 5. Allow perimenopause to take its course:

The fifth ingredient that can be added to the mixture for a positive perimenopause experience is for the woman to simply **allow the perimenopause process to take its course**. Just as adolescence and the childbirth process posed its physical and psychological challenges, so too will perimenopause. A woman needs to know that it is *okay* to have an unpleasant day here and there, which can sometimes be more often than not. Most of us, in Western societies anyway, are probably going to experience some negative perimenopausal signs; remember that almost 85% of American women experiencing perimenopause will have *some* negative signs.

## 6. Keep looking ahead:

No matter how bad things get, always look ahead to better days. Remember that most negative perimenopausal signs are only temporary. They will pass. And, as mentioned earlier, most women feel better overall anyway after menopause, so there is something to look forward to. Keep looking ahead.

## 7. Assume and maintain a positive attitude *throughout* the perimenopause process:

The seventh approach to meeting perimenopause optimistically involves acquiring and maintaining a **positive attitude throughout the perimenopause process**. As simple as this may sound, it can become tremendously hard keeping a positive attitude in the midst of negative perimenopausal signs and other external events that may be placing many extra demands and pressures on the woman. But, a positive attitude can do wonders for both physical and mental health. It has been demonstrated time and time again in the medical field that when patients maintain a positive attitude, they fare much better in their treatment plans than patients who don't have a positive attitude. Patients who have a positive attitude pre and post-op have a faster recovery from surgery and experience less pain, burns tend to heal more quickly, there is an increased resistance to arthritis, a decreased incidence of heart disease,[162] and there is even improved immune system functioning. Women with a positive state of mind cope more effectively during pregnancy, which could be a deterrent to adverse birth outcomes.[163] Furthermore, according to a study conducted at Yale (July 29, 2002), individuals with a positive attitude tend to live longer than individuals who fear and dread aging (7.5 years longer). Individuals who keep an optimistic attitude toward the aging process appear to have more determination to remain alive and they also appear to prevent and avoid increased stress levels that can accompany negative feelings about the aging process itself.[164] It has also been suggested that a positive attitude has *more* of an influence on a longer life than a low cholesterol level or low blood pressure.[165] It's amazing, isn't it, the power of the mind? There is such an intense mind-body association in overall health, that a new branch of medicine, psychoneuroimmunology, has been developed to examine this very connection between mental attitude and health.[166]

## 8. Assume and maintain a positive perception *of* the perimenopause process:

Following the above mentioned perimenopausal management strategy, it has been theorized that **the unpleasant signs of perimenopause may actually be more pronounced, or may even have an increased chance of occurrence if the woman attaches a negative meaning** to the perimenopause process itself.[167] As with *any* life experience that is internalized negatively, the individual will probably have more difficulty with the experience. The psychological impact of perimenopause (and finally menopause) is related to what the entire process implies to the woman. A society's established views are extremely important, but equally if not more important, is a woman's own personal perception of perimenopause in determining the meaning of menopause.[168] By greeting perimenopause with a smile, a woman can actually minimize or even prevent negative signs.

Since menopause is viewed differently in each society, the menopause process is culturally a very varied experience. Unfortunately, our American society has historically conditioned women (and everyone else around them) to dread and fear menopause. Remember that in the not so distant past, menopause was a forbidden subject that was never even discussed. A more optimistic conditioning process will probably take *years* of evolvement before our society as a whole views menopause in a more positive way. And, I am hoping that this book will make some contribution in leading the way to a more enthusiastic view of the menopause experience. Let's remind ourselves again that the passage through perimenopause is simply the beginning of another chapter in life. It is a milestone to be celebrated.

## 9. External events may be responsible for an increase in the occurrence and/or the severity of negative perimenopausal signs:

It has been postulated that the overall **perimenopause progression is quite dependent on the context and the external circumstances occurring** in a woman's life at the time of perimenopause. Unfortunately, we don't have much power over the timing of or the gravity of external events in life. And, the more stressors/pressures/challenges that are confronting a woman in her life concurrently with perimenopause, the more pessimistically she will experience this particular time of life. It has been proven, for example, that stress has been linked with an increase in the incidence and/or the intensity of hot flashes.[169] This negativity would most likely develop with any circumstance in life that presented simultaneously with other undesirable or unexpected pressures/challenges/stressors that posed additional stresses, demands, and/or responsibilities on an individual. Psychologically speaking, the main event (perimenopause) becomes associated with the negative peripheral events. Additional outside responsibilities and/or demands can place extra burdens on the perimenopausal woman at a time when she really requires her energies to be directed toward her own metamorphosis.

## 10. Don't put perimenopause needs *last* on the list of priorities:

Like so many other middle-aged women, I had *sooo* many stressors present at this point in my life. I lost my job in an economy that was very sluggishly recovering, resulting in few good available jobs and we were quickly slipping into a serious financial bind because of the drastic drop in income. My son was entering adolescence. And, my mother was a geriatric of 86 who's health was beginning to deteriorate. And, even though she was very independent and lived on her own, I worried about her. Now, any *one* of these external events happening independently would have been plenty for one person to handle, but *all* of them occurring simultaneously was *very* disturbing and *incredibly* intimidating. Not that perimenopause was to blame for any one of these peripheral concerns in my life, but it did seem like the personal negative perimenopausal signs that I was experiencing were just an additional encumbrance that I had to endure on top of all of my other concerns. It was funny because I could manage the external issues somehow, but I felt that the perimenopausal signs that I was experiencing were just plain bothersome and disruptive. And, I felt that perimenopause couldn't have entered my life at a worse time! There were just way too many things happening *to* me and *around* me at the same time.

And then one day out of the blue, a very remarkable thought came to me: *Maybe a personal paradigm shift was in order here. I should be tending to my own internal perimenopausal issues with priority.* Instead, up to this point, every*one* else and every*thing* else around me took precedence while my own physical and mental issues took a back seat. Generally speaking, women are nurturers who tend to put their own wants and needs on the back burner anyway. So...perimenopause would not be any different in that a woman's own needs would come second to her other responsibilities. However, maybe a change in thinking is indeed overdue. Women need to learn to tend to their own personal priorities and not ignore their own needs whatever they may be, e.g. more sleep, a day off, a day away, peaceful time, exercise, a cup of tea, etc.

## 11. Manage and/or delegate external responsibilities and demands:

In an attempt to prevent external pressures from negatively impacting the time of perimenopause, a woman may have to empower others to perform certain personal or business tasks or duties that may be placing extra demands on her at this time. By delegating certain responsibilities to others, a woman can free herself of some of the burden of unrealistic and untimely demands. Unfortunately, delegating is not an easy task in and of itself for women in that women have historically been conditioned to assume an "I'll do it all" position, which has in turn put excessive and unreasonable expectations on many American females. But, whether it is in the workplace or in the household, handing over some burdensome responsibilities may become a necessary part of life now.

## 12. Withhold public displays of perimenopausal emotionality in the workplace:

No matter how difficult it might be, a woman must *not ever* show sudden emotionality (weeping, snapping, yelling, expressing anger, etc.) related to perimenopause in the workplace! As I mentioned earlier, I heard *so* many negative comments, from men and women alike, about my previous boss lady who cried frequently and could not seem to control her emotions in the business setting. Our society, in general, has a tendency to support a more cheerful attitude toward problems and even prefers silence to emotional outbursts. And, following this societal norm, most American work environments are designed in a way that discourages any display of negative emotion. If a woman does *not* want to commit career suicide, she should hold back any display of negative emotions related to perimenopause in the workplace. If a woman feels a "perimenopausal moment" approaching, she should excuse herself and immediately remove herself from that meeting/interaction/confrontation/etc. She can go to the ladies room, go outside and take some deep breaths, take a quick walk, use mental imagery, *whatever* she has to do to separate herself from that emotional ignition switch, she should absolutely do it. And, she should be prepared to do this without hesitation should the need arise.

## 13. Talk, talk, talk:

Another mental management strategy in confronting perimenopause successfully is to **talk about it**!!! They say that experience is the best teacher and it probably is. The perimenopausal woman can gain such valuable information and insight into perimenopause by simply talking with other women who have experienced it themselves or have known other women whom have experienced it. As mentioned earlier, sharing stories is integral to each and every individual's development. By discussing, sharing, inquiring, and listening, a woman can educate herself by extrapolating bits and pieces of others' stories to better identify with and understand her own perimenopause experience. I personally had a tough time trying to get other women to open up and discuss their experiences with me which led me to believe that even though our culture *is* very slowly progressing beyond old standards and traditions involving menopause, we still have a lot of work to do in getting women to open up and talk about the menopause process. Any shame, embarrassment, or awkwardness is completely unfounded, nonsensical, and truly a thing of the past. The silence and resulting mystery that once surrounded the menopause transition needs to disappear with this new era that has just begun. We must embrace this new millennium with all of its opportunities for knowledge and information and strive for positive changes in women's health and well being. Furthermore, we *must* learn to free ourselves from self-imposed restrictions and past ignorance.

Additionally, a woman who **shares and communicates** her perimenopausal discomforts and/or concerns with loved ones can also ease a great deal of tension, especially in the home. If others are made aware of certain physical and psychological signs or emotions that are present in the perimenopausal woman, "Oh, that is how she feels today," then loved ones will most likely be much more compassionate and helpful. Keep in mind that there is inconsistency and unpredictability in most of the perimenopausal signs that appear. So…if loved ones are cognizant of the woman's feelings and physical status, then they will probably be more empathetic and understanding. Many women are hesitant to share their feelings with others and this may complicate already strained relationships when loved ones are left in the dark guessing about the perimenopausal woman's extreme, unusual, or unexpected behavior.

Moreover, by talking with a spouse, a loved one, a friend, or anyone who is willing to be an attentive listener about the way she is feeling, a perimenopausal woman can alleviate some of the pent-up emotion she may be experiencing.

## 14. Clean out the closet:

Another approach to managing perimenopause successfully is to get rid of mental garbage. The musician known as Eminem recently released a song titled, *Cleaning out the closet*. The incredibly powerful and moving lyrics refer to the necessity of getting all of the heavy, burdening mental baggage (skeletons, trash or whatever) out from behind closed doors and into the open to face it and deal with it to be able to move on in life happily. For Eminem, it was confronting the fact that his father abandoned the family when Em was only an infant. And, if it wasn't enough for a young, innocent child to have to grow up fatherless in this world, he had to deal with the horrific and ruthless way his mother treated him throughout his childhood.

To successfully move forward in life, it is probably best for women to go ahead and "clean out their closets" at this mid-point in life—at least get the garbage out from behind closed doors. If that means visiting a psychologist, then so be it. It can become difficult for us to process all of the complexities of this life by ourselves and outside professional assistance from a psychologist, psychiatrist, psychoanalyst, etc. may be very helpful. Also, dealing with the baggage now, at the approximate halfway point in life, eliminates the need to have to deal with it toward the end of the lifespan, when it becomes much more difficult to deal with.

Obviously, some people like Eminem (who is only in his twenties at the time I am writing this), realize that they need an early closet sweep. But, many of us go through our daily routines well into our forties and fifties not giving this stuff a second thought. We are much too busy and/or unwilling to even look *in* the closet, much less clean it out! And, in reality, any dissatisfaction, unhappiness, disappointment, and/or frustration with the past only compounds any negative perimenopausal signs a woman may be experiencing. So, a thorough closet cleaning (at least getting the stuff out into the open) becomes essential to the perimenopausal woman in assisting her to achieve well health and happiness and in helping her to move on in life emotionally healthy, minus all the oppressive baggage.

## 15. Come to terms with past life outcomes:

Following a closet sweep, a woman needs to **come to terms with past life outcomes**. Once the issues are out of the closet and exposed, it then becomes easy to confront them. At this approximate mid-point in the lifespan, most of us, men included, become introspective. That is, we seem to reflect upon our previous life choices and we evaluate the outcomes. This is similar to working on a project that is half completed, say painting a room with a faux finish technique, and we take a moment to step back to thoughtfully and carefully review our work to decipher whether we want to continue with the same approach to finishing the project or follow another more appropriate strategy to completion. Likewise, if we are really not satisfied with the person we have become, with the education we have received, with the financial situation we have created, with the job choices that have been made, with our relationship selections, etc., there is bound to be inner turmoil. Let's be realistic, *few* of us have had a life where *everything* has gone our way. And, at times, some obstacles or other complications that may have arisen may have made our choices that much more complex. We have all made choices that may *not* have been the same choices we would make again.

If we look at this mid-life appraisal in a positive way, this mid-life self assessment actually allows us to step back and review past choices and outcomes at the approximate halfway mark in our lives and to modify, change, and/or update our progress. Even if we have made really poor choices in the past and our lives have not unfolded as we planned, we still have the second half of life to fix it. Or, even if we thought we made really great choices in the past, but the outcomes were not as positive as we planned, we still have time to correct them. Or, even if we have made excellent choices and the outcomes were very successful, there is always room for improvement in some area of life. What a *disaster* it would be not performing this mid-life evaluation and to continue on the same unproductive, destructive, inefficient, disorganized, unhappy, or unhealthy path through life. Most importantly though, we cannot relive the past, so most of us need to come to terms with and somehow resolve previous decisions and/or outcomes that have negatively impacted us and then make the necessary adjustments.

## 16. Serve as a role model to society:

It is really important for American women today that this society starts assuming a more positive attitude toward the menopause metamorphosis and starts honoring it. As mentioned previously, a woman's cultural standards are *extremely* important in her journey down the road of perimenopause. One American woman can make a difference and start this ball rolling simply by becoming a role model for others. By possessing the knowledge, positive attitude, patience, openness, and grace during the perimenopause process, she can become a positive example to the rest of society.

# 9

# *The Final Metamorphosis*

I would like to take the opportunity in this final chapter to share with you some personal perimenopause thoughts and events that I myself experienced while developing this project and then conclude with some final thoughts.

At the age of forty-five, I first realized that my final metamorphosis had begun. I never thought I would make it this far and yet here I was in middle age experiencing the last sexual transition we call menopause. In the very beginning of the process, when I first sat down and started writing this book, I was experiencing horrific migraine headaches on a regular basis. This actually slowed the book's progress down as on some days when I had a debilitating headache, I just couldn't face the computer. However, not only was I entering perimenopause, but I had just been dismissed from a job that I really loved due to a downsizing, I had a son approaching adolescence, and my 86 year old mother was having some health troubles. As stated earlier in the book, oftentimes there are *so* many other significant life events occurring in mid-life simultaneously with perimenopause that I was quite understandably feeling overwhelmed. Not only had I lost my job, but the repercussions of that event left me with serious financial problems. And, not only was my son adolescing, but he was having difficulty in his identity search. Finally, not only was my mother facing health issues, but she had *three* operations in a matter of twelve months! I had other peripheral concerns as well, but these three main events were the most significant and affected me the most. I also noticed that my normal behavior was altered at the very onset of perimeno-pause, i.e. I was irritable, impatient, depressed, and overly anxious. And, many days, I just felt exhausted, really exhausted. At the time I first sat down and started to write this book, I was only vaguely aware of what was changing my entire personality, and I knew that it was very important for me to find out exactly what it was.

With the development of this project, being able to identify the exact cause of my aching joints and my changed behaviors was such an incredible relief. Who would have ever thought that hormones would be to blame? The knowledge that I was able to access and assemble into this book through the many mediums available today has helped me substantially in traveling through perimenopause. I am now very aware of what is happening to me physiologically, physically, and psychologically. And, now I am quite confident that I can manage the negative aspects of perimenopause without difficulty and I look forward to the positive aspects of this major life experience. The psychological and physical jackpot at the end of the of perimenopause rainbow are rewards that I welcome. For example, since that time almost two years ago, when I first sat down to work on this book, the headaches that I experienced on a regular basis have subsided drastically, and I only have a headache here and there. That in itself is a great relief. The joint aches that I was experiencing have also decreased considerably. I started taking calcium supplements (ask your health care professional, pharmacist, or health food store/vitamin store representative for the exact dosage for your age) and I also started working out with dumbbells routinely. Remember that weight bearing exercises can strengthen bones.

Even though my patience level remains altered at this time, I am aware of it therefore allowing me to control it. I am consciously aware of my feelings and behaviors all the time now. I try to be especially aware of others' feelings if I am having a "perimenopausal moment". The depressed moments have tapered off too. One positive element in reducing my depression I am sure has to do with the fact that I finally found that my passion in life was to be an author and since making that revelation and writing this book, I have become extremely satisfied with my life. I believe that I have finally found my niche. I still have down days, but nothing like the days in the beginning of perimenopause. Furthermore, time has moved on and I have (1) survived losing my job, (2) lived through my son's hormones, and (3) my mother is now healthy again going on 88 years of age. Life really does get better!

I have also conducted a closet sweep here in the middle of my life, just like Eminem. Unfortunately, I waited well into my forties to perform the sweep. But, I figure that it is better than doing the cleaning somewhere in my eighties when forty more years have passed and forty more years of clutter has accumulated in the closet. I am still processing some of the garbage, and it is a gradual process, but nevertheless it is out in the open (if only in my mind).

Additionally, I should mention that I am a pet lover and I have three dogs. One is from the Humane Society, one was given to us from an expanding family with six children that couldn't deal with the needs of a pedigree dog anymore, and one was purchased from a breeder as a baby. Each of these dogs is special in her own way and each dog heals me on a daily basis. These dogs have really helped me travel down the road of perimenopause and they are always there for me whether I have a good day or a bad day. Pets are great therapy for anyone.

With the onset of perimenopause, there are the common presenting physical characteristics of the process. Even if perimenopause is only a temporary event, the hormonal fluctuations and/or declines can easily thrust a woman into not feeling like her typical self as I can testify to. Perimenopause may appear as a burden, problem, inconvenience (haven't got time for the pain), or aggravation in the midst of especially busy and demanding schedules today. When in fact, a woman needs to learn to be attentive to her own physical needs and address any negative perimenopausal signs. Equally, if not more important, are the psychological influences of perimenopause. There are mental inconsistencies including irritability, mood swings, anxiety, depression, feelings of helplessness, feelings of worthlessness, and/or a decrease or change in cognitive performance. A woman's behavior can be affected on every level during perimenopause. And, a perimenopausal woman must not only face these inconsistencies, but she must also manage their sometimes sudden appearance. However, perimenopause can become the catalyst for tremendous psychological growth and potential in that it forces a woman to take a long, hard look at herself, i.e. her lifestyle, her relationships, her career, her education, her finances, her assets, her eating and exercise habits, and her life in general up to this point. She still has approximately another half of the lifespan to change, modify, and meet her goals. Remember that I found my own passion of writing at the age of forty-five. I can really say that perimenopause has changed my life forever in a very positive way!

Unfortunately, many women still approach this phase of life stumbling through it uninformed, misinformed, confused, uncomfortable, embarrassed, self-conscious, and somewhat clueless about what to expect. But, by educating herself, by exposing herself to as much written and verbal information as possible, and by communicating about the perimenopause process (sharing, extracting stories from other women, etc.), a woman can sail through the entire perimenopause event feeling empowered and with dignity because she has prepared herself with the most powerful perimenopause management tool available—**knowledge**.

From my experience with other women, i.e. other women lacking openness about their own perimenopause, there is clearly a tremendous gap in verbal communication that exists between women regarding the perimenopause process. Women remain uncomfortable talking about menopause. I hope that this book has helped to alleviate some of the awkwardness that women feel sharing their stories. Perimenopause is a unique female life event, similar to the motherhood experience that *must* start bringing women closer together. And, from my research revealing that there was an even greater gap in the written psychological material available concerning perimenopause, I hope that this book has served as an initiator to filling in that gap.

Finally, it has been almost two years since I first started this project and I must say that it has been an *amazing* and *enlightening* journey. I have tried to pull together as much information as I could gather about the perimenopause process and put it into one concise resource for women to be able to refer to. I have tried to keep the book to the point and short enough so as not to overwhelm an already overwhelmed population of women! My own perimenopause metamorphosis would not have been as positive as it has been so far, if not for this project. I want to thank each and every one of you who read this book for you have opened up a whole new world to me; A world of allowing me to share my thoughts, feelings, knowledge, and research with you. I truly appreciate this opportunity. And, I wish for you a successful passage through perimenopause!

# Glossary of Terms ☺

**Activities of Daily Living (ADL's)**: The activities we perform normally in daily living including self-care (eating, bathing, dressing, grooming), work, domestic chores, exercise, and leisure activities.[170]

**Adaptation**: (1) An alteration/adjustment in structure or habits, often hereditary, by which an individual or species improves its condition in relationship to its environment.[171] (2) The adjustment of an organism to its environment, or the process by which the organism enhances fitness.[172]

**Arthralgia**: Pain in a joint or joints.[173]

**Fluctuation**: Alternate rise and fall; to vary irregularly.[174]

**Gestational Diabetes**: A form of diabetes mellitus appearing during pregnancy (gestation) in a woman who previously did not have diabetes. It is usually noticed between the 24th and 28th week of the pregnancy. Blood glucose levels typically return to normal after the baby is born.[175,176]

**Homeostasis**: (1) The maintenance of relatively stable internal physiological conditions in higher animals.[177] (2) A tendency toward stability in the normal body states (internal environment) of the organism.[178]

**Neuroendocrine**: The interactions between the nervous system and the endocrine system.[179]

**National Institutes of Health (NIH)**: Founded in 1887, the NIH (comprising 27 separate Institutes and Centers) is one of the world's foremost medical research centers and Federal focal point for medical research in the U.S. The goal of NIH research is to acquire new knowledge to help prevent, detect, diagnose, and treat disease and disability.[180]

**Natural or Bioidentical Hormones (BHRT)**: Are synthesized from natural plant substances to be identical in structure and function to the hormones the body produced naturally pre-menopause.[181]

**Pre-eclampsia**: A toxic condition of late pregnancy characterized by sudden hypertension (high blood pressure), generalized edema (fluid retention), excessive weight gain, severe headache, visual disturbances, and proteinuria (protein in the urine). It typically occurs after the 20th week of the pregnancy.[182,183]

**Sociocultural**: Of, relating to, or involving a combination of social and cultural factors.[184]

**Xenoestrogens**: (Xenobiotics) Are petrochemicals that are found in solvents, pesticides, herbicides, adhesives, plastic products, and artificial fabrics. These compounds are toxic; they can disturb our hormonal balance and can increase our cancer risk.[185]

# References

[1] www.mayoclinic.com

[2] On Death and Dying. Elisabeth Kubler-Ross, Touchstone, New York, NY 1969, 1997

[3] Healthy Aging, Healthy Treatment, The Impact of Telling Stories. Thomas H. Peake, Praeger Publishing, Wesport, CT 1998, p.76

[4] Healthy Aging, Healthy Treatment, The Impact of Telling Stories. Thomas H. Peake, Praeger Publishing, Wesport, CT 1998, p.2

[5] dictionary.reference.com

[6] dictionary.reference.com

[7] www.healthywomen.org

[8] www.healthywomen.org

[9] www.earlymenopause.com

[10] www.earlymenopause.com

[11] www.earlymenopause.com

[12] content.health.msn.com

[13] www.psychologytoday.com; New Research on Menopause, Richard Lovett, Ph.D., May 2, 2003

[14] www.psychologytoday.com; New Research on Menopause, Richard Lovett, Ph.D., May 2, 2003

[15] www.menopause.org

[16] www.menopause.org

[17] www.menopause.org

[18] Aging Research Center (ARC), www.arclab.org

[19] www.womenshealthamerica.com

[20] American Fitness, March 2001, Carol Krucoff, Mitchell Krucoff

[21] www.plannedparenthood.org

[22] www.mayoclinic.com

[23] The Foundation for Better Healthcare at www.fbhc.org

[24] www.naturalhealthweb.com

[25] www.psychologytoday.com; New Research on Menopause, Richard Lovett, Ph.D., May 2, 2003

[26] cnn.com

[27] www.geocities.com

[28] www.geocities.com

[29] Hawkes K, O'Connell JF, Jones NGB. Hadza women's time allocation, off-spring provisioning, and the evolution of long postmenopausal life spans. *Current Anthropology* 38(4), 551–77, 1997.

[30] www.myhealthspan.com

[31] www.myhealthspan.com

[32] www.kmcnetwork.healthwords.com

[33] www.nof.org (The National Osteoporosis Foundation)

[34] www.nof.org (The National Osteoporosis Foundation)

[35] www.mayoclinic.com

[36] www.menopausecanada.com

[37] www.texmed.org

[38] www.fda.gov

[39] www.fda.gov

[40] www.healthywomen.org

[41] www.project-aware.org

[42] www.medicineau.net.au (Medicine Australia)

[43] www.womhealth.org.au

[44] www.womhealth.org.au

[45] www.womhealth.org.au

[46] www.womhealth.org.au

[47] www.thefreedictionary.com

[48] www.menopause-online.com

[49] www.menopause-online.com

[50] www.menopause-online.com

[51] Woods NF, Mitchell ES, Patterns of depressed mood in midlife women: Observations from the Seattle Midlife Women's Health Study, Res Nurs Health, 1996:19:111–123

[52] www.menopause-online.com

[53] Psychology Today, March-April 2003, Richard A. Lovett

[54] www.4woman.gov

[55] National Institutes of Health, 3–29–2000

[56] www.medicineau.net.au (Medicine Australia)

[57] www.ucsf.edu

[58] www.cwhn.ca (The Canadian Women's Health Network)

[59] www.womentowomen.com

[60] www.cdc.gov (Centers for Disease Control and Prevention)

[61] www.dvmen.org (Domestic Violence Studies; supported and maintained by the Equal Justice Foundation)

[62] www.dvmen.org (Domestic Violence Studies; supported and maintained by the Equal Justice Foundation), Stets and Straus (1989)

[63] www.dvmen.org (Domestic Violence Studies; supported and maintained by the Equal Justice Foundation), Stets and Straus (1989)

[64] www.preventelderabuse.org

[65] www.cancer.gov

[66] <u>What Your Doctor May Not Tell you about Menopause</u>, John R. Lee, M.D. & Virginia Hopkins, Warner Books, 2004

[67] www.sleepfoundation.org

[68] www.menopause-online.com

[69] www.menopause-online.com

[70] www.menopause-online.com

[71] www.menopause-online.com

[72] www.springboard4health.com

[73] www.springboard4health.com

[74] www.plannedparenthood.org

[75] www.mypleasure.com

[76] National Institutes of Health

[77] www.mayoclinic.com

[78] www.4woman.gov

[79] discovery.com

[80] www.healthcentral.com

[81] www.medscan.com

[82] www.medscan.com

[83] www.womenwithhairloss.com

[84] www.healthsquare.com

[85] www.more-selfesteem.com

[86] www.coping.org

[87] www.coping.org

[88] www.coping.org

[89] www.coping.org

[90] www.coping.com

[91] www.dictionary.reference.com

[92] www.womensmedia.com

[93] www.4woman.gov

[94] www.bbc.co.uk

[95] www.healthwatcher.net

[96] www.healthwatcher.net

[97] www.sirc.org (Social Issues Research Centre)

[98] www.healthsquare.com

[99] American Fitness, March 2001, Carol Krucoff, Mitchell Krucoff

[100] www.cnn.com

[101] www.womenshealth.about.com

[102] www.womenshealth.about.com

[103] www.blackwomenshealth.com

[104] www.niapublications.org

[105] www.upi.com

[106] www.4woman.gov (The National Women's Health Information Center)

[107] www.4woman.gov (The National Women's Health Information Center)

[108] www.4woman.gov (The National Women's Health Information Center)

[109] www.4woman.gov (The National Women's Health Information Center)

[110] www.4woman.gov (The National Women's Health Information Center)

[111] www.4woman.gov (The National Women's Health Information Center)

[112] www.ijpc.com (International Journal of Pharmaceutical Compounding, Vol. 5, No.5, Sept-Oct 2001)

[113] www.thenaturalhuman.com

[114] www.ijpc.com (International Journal of Pharmaceutical Compounding, Vol. 5, No.5, Sept-Oct 2001)

[115] www.thecompounder.com

[116] www.project-aware.org (Association of Women for the Advancement of Research and Education)

[117] www.healthandnutrition.co.uk

[118] www.project-aware.org

[119] www.prevention.com

[120] www.naturebasket.com

[121] www.healthlink.mcw.edu

[122] www.healthandnutrition.co.uk

[123] www.healthandnutrition.co.uk

[124] www.healthandnutrition.co.uk

[125] www.womenshealth.about.com

[126] www.project-aware.org

[127] www.healthandnutrition.co.uk

[128] www.lifefitness.com

[129] www.womenshealth.about.com

130 www.menopauserx.com

131 www.americanyogaassociation.com

132 www.holistic-online.com

133 www.indiamedicalinfo.com

134 www.naturalhealthweb.com

135 www.indiamedicalinfo.com

136 www.indiamedicalinfo.com

137 www.naturalhealthweb.com

138 www.naturalhealthweb.com

139 www.chclibrary.org

140 www.chclibrary.org

141 www.holistic-online.com

142 www.alternative-therapies.com

143 www.cwhn.ca (The Canadian Women's Health Network)

144 www.cwhn.ca (The Canadian Women's Health Network)

145 www.arhp.org

146 www.healthsquare.com

147 www.bbc.co.uk

148 www.justaddmilk.ca, *Demystifying Menopause*

149 www.mothersover40.com

150 www.betterhealth.vic.gov.au (Better Health Channel in association with The Australian Psychological Society, Ltd.)

151 www.betterhealth.vic.gov.au (Better Health Channel in association with The Australian Psychological Society, Ltd.)

152 middleage.org

153 Journal of Family Practice, March 2002, Linda French

154 www.nhlbi.nih.gov, National Institutes of Health,Chapter 4—*Sociocultural Issues in Menopause,* by Aila Collins, Ph.D.

155 www.menopause-online.com

156 Marcha Flint, 1982, Male and female menopause: A cultural put-on.

157 Marcha Flint, 1982, Male and female menopause: A cultural put-on.

158 www.upi.com

159 www.nhlbi.nih.gov

160 www.nhlbi.nih.gov

161 news.bbc.co.uk

162 Hopkins' Center for Health Promotion study

163 Journal of Health Psychology, November 2000

164 Journal of Personality and Positive Psychology, August 2002

[165] Journal of Personality and Positive Psychology, August 2002

[166] Journal of Personality and Positive Psychology, August 2002

[167] Menopause: The Journal of The North American Menopause Society, Vol. 10, No. 2, pp. 179–187

[168] www.nhlbi.nih.gov, National Institutes of Health, Chapter 4—*Sociocultural Issues in Menopause,* by Aila Collins, Ph.D.

[169] Holisticonline.com

[170] medical-dictionary.com

[171] www.dictionary.com

[172] medical-dictionary.com

[173] www.dictionary.com

[174] www.dictionary.com

[175] www.medterms.com

[176] medical-dictionary.com

[177] www2.merriam-webster.com

[178] medical-dictionary.com

[179] www.medterms.com

[180] www.nih.gov

[181] www.springboard4health.com

[182] medical-dictionary.com

[183] www2.merriam-webster.com

[184] www2.merriam-webster.com

[185] www.menopause-natural.com

# *Additional Perimenopause Resources*

**The National Women's Health Information Center** (**NWHIC**) is a service of the Office on Women's Health in the Department of Health of Human Services that has a web site and toll free information center providing free, reliable, health information for women. "The Federal Government Source for Women's Health Information".
**www.4women.gov or 1-800-994-WOMAN**

**Project Aware (Association of Women for the Advancement of Research and Education)** is a "website by women, for women, offering objective and comprehensive health information, especially related to menopause, perimenopause, and post menopause".
**www.project-aware.org**

**National Women's Health Resource Center, Inc. (NWHRC)** is a non-profit organization that "helps women make informed decisions about their health".
**www.healthywomen.org or 1-877-986-9472**

**Menopause Online** is an online site that "provides up-to-date information to make the menopausal transition smooth".
**www.menopause-online.com**

**The North American Menopause Society (NAMS)** is a "nonprofit scientific organization devoted to promoting women's health and quality of life through an understanding of menopause".
**www.menopause.org**

**Coping.org (Tools for Coping with Life's Stressors)** is an online site that assists individuals in "coping with a variety of life's stressors".
**www.coping.org**

978-0-595-34624-0
0-595-34624-3